Praise for *The Practice of the Yoga Sutra: Sadhana Pada*

The *Yoga Sutra* of Patanjali offers a path through which practitioners may experience deep personal transformation on their journey through life. Unfortunately, this transformational potential is often inaccessible to the modern student—perhaps because of the text's antiquity and terse sutra style of composition.

In his extraordinary work, *The Practice of the Yoga Sutra: Sadhana Pada*, Pandit Rajmani reveals and explains hidden teachings and practices, transforming what may seem an obscure or even academic treatise into a meaningful and vitally relevant manual for conscious living. This book is a rare gift and a must-read for all serious students of yoga.

—Gary Kraftsow, MA, founder of the American Viniyoga Institute and author of *Yoga for Transformation*

In my opinion, Panditji's lucid new commentary on the *Yoga Sutra* will become the gold standard for commentaries on this important scripture. As was the case with his first volume, *The Secret of the Yoga Sutra*, on the "Samadhi Pada," the newly released *The Practice of the Yoga Sutra*, on the "Sadhana Pada" is immensely inspiring. It is remarkably detailed and scholarly, yet at the same time, accessible to the mainstream reader—a feat not easy to pull off. Once I began reading this new effort, I simply could not put it down. Even now, it sits next to my bed for rereading and study. Every student of yoga should be happy to have this wonderful new guide.

—Stephen Cope, senior scholar-in-residence at the Kripalu Center for Yoga and Health, and author of *Yoga and the Quest for the True Self* and *The Wisdom of Yoga*

In *The Practice of the Yoga Sutra: Sadhana Pada*, Pandit Rajmani Tigunait presents an elegant and clear interpretation of yoga practice from the perspective of Sri Vidya, a school of thought that celebrates how spirit infuses all aspects of human experience and the world.

All readers will enjoy this valuable volume: The beginner will be introduced to the basic practices of yoga, including control of breath and foundational ethics. Those with more experience with yoga will benefit from the grammatical and philosophical analyses and the appendixes in the back that facilitate easy chanting and offer detailed information on practices found in the Himalayan Tradition.

Sadhana Pada explains the role of karma in determining the human condition and provides a threefold and eightfold path toward freedom. This book makes a superb introduction to the principles and practices of yoga.

—Christopher Key Chapple, Doshi Professor of Indic and Comparative Theology and director of the Master of Arts in Yoga Studies Program at Loyola Marymount University

The *Yoga Sutra* of Patanjali is receiving much new attention in the yoga world today but remains largely misunderstood and misinterpreted, with its broader connections ignored. In this context, it is heartening to see a helpful, yet profound and authentic, presentation of the text by Pandit Rajmani Tigunait.

Pandit Rajmani has provided a comprehensive, clear, and accessible commentary on the second part of the *Yoga Sutra*, the "Sadhana Pada," that teaches the prime structure of yoga practice leading to samadhi. His approach is experiential, not speculative or academic. His connection of the *Yoga Sutra* with both Vedanta and Tantra is notable. His discussion of the main aspects of yoga practice puts them in the proper perspective for the serious practitioner to follow and apply.

His series on the *Yoga Sutra* overall is excellent and should be carefully studied by all yoga students who aspire to connect with the deeper tradition behind yoga.

—David Frawley, DLitt, Padma Bhushan, director of the American Institute of Vedic Studies

As I initially began to skim this remarkable commentary, I found myself slowing down, highlighting many sentences, and personally reflecting on illuminating passages. I've read multiple commentaries on the *Yoga Sutra*, but nothing as deeply educational and truly inspiring as this.

—John Kepner, executive director of The International Association of Yoga Therapists

Pandit Rajmani Tigunait's illuminating commentary on "Sadhana Pada," the second chapter of the *Yoga Sutra*, is a must-read for all yoga students. His wisdom, knowledge, and direct experience, born from his personal practice and dedicated study, infuse every chapter. He offers readers profound insights into the practice of yoga that get to the heart of the matter: how we reduce pain and suffering and awaken our joy, innate beauty, and creativity. He leaves us no doubt about the possibility of success when we systematically follow the instructions he clearly elucidates. This book holds the keys to a visionary approach to life—one where we collectively take self-responsibility and awaken to our divinity.

—Kia Miller, founder of Radiant Body Yoga

Many of us come to yoga as outsiders exploring an exotic foreign tradition. Pandit Tigunait is an insider, a direct disciple of one of the most influential yoga masters of the past century. I can hardly imagine anyone more qualified to introduce Western readers to the *Yoga Sutra* as it has actually been understood by yoga adepts.

The Practice of the Yoga Sutra is brimming with unique insights, not only from classical sources like Vyasa's authoritative commentary, but also from Pandit Tigunait's own Sri Vidya lineage—one of the most fascinating and esoteric of India's tantric traditions.

This modern classic challenges readers to take their spiritual practice to a whole new level. Very highly recommended.

—Linda Johnsen, MS, author of *Lost Masters: Rediscovering the Mysticism of the Ancient Greek Philosophers*

Patanjali's *Yoga Sutra* is so concise and so dense with meaning that it requires expert interpretation. Hundreds of commentaries have been rendered over the centuries, and yet Pandit Tigunait has given us something new. By focusing exclusively on the second pada, he examines the *Sutra's* most applicable wisdom, and by expanding on the commentary of the great sage Vyasa, he injects that practical information with penetrating insight. This most welcome addition to the literature of modern yoga should be relished by both students of the philosophy and practitioners of the precious eight-limbed path.

—Philip Goldberg, author of *American Veda: From Emerson and the Beatles to Yoga and Meditation, How Indian Spirituality Changed the West*

It is impossible to overstate what an immense contribution is made *The Practice of the Yoga Sutra*. Pandit Rajmani Tigunait's commentary is a revelation, providing insights into the hidden teachings of the second chapter of the *Yoga Sutra*. From time immemorial, the guidance of a true master has been considered essential to understand and to practice yoga in a way that leads to its ultimate reward—lasting freedom and fulfillment. Thankfully, Pandit Rajmani's wisdom illuminates these pages, decoding everything from the practical to the most exalted, from how to practice on and off your mat, to explaining the otherwise unexplainable mysteries of consciousness. Read it to create your own path to enlightenment.

—Rod Stryker, founder of ParaYoga and author of *The Four Desires: Creating a Life of Purpose, Happiness, Prosperity, and Freedom*

Pandit Rajmani Tigunait takes the reader on a transformative journey in *The Practice of the Yoga Sutra: Sadhana Pada*. Both new students and those who have traversed this territory before will find vistas of fresh inspiration drawn from the well of ancient Vedic wisdom and the depths of Panditji's decades of sadhana. That meeting place of ancient wisdom and modern-day sadhana offers the reader a life-affirming vision like no other: We are the highest expression of our creator's joy, and we are destined to experience that joy.

—Yogacharya Ellen Grace O'Brian, spiritual director of the Center for Spiritual Enlightenment and author of *Living the Eternal Way: Spiritual Meaning and Practice in Daily Life*

Pandit Rajmani has infused light and life into the minds of sincere seekers with his commentary on "Sadhana Pada." This book is written in a simple format, yet it does not compromise the essence of the subject discussed—yoga.

—Indu Arora, director of Yoga Sadhna and author of *Mudra: The Sacred Secret*

What a pleasure to see a fresh translation of the most practical chapter in the *Yoga Sutra*, translated eloquently by a true Sanskrit scholar and yoga adept. Pandit Rajmani's rendering is authentic, sensible, understandable, and comprehensive. I highly recommend it.

—Nicolai Bachman, MA, teacher of Sanskrit and yoga philosophy, and author of *The Language of Yoga* and *The Path of the Yoga Sutras*

The Practice *of the* Yoga Sutra

Books in This Series

The Secret of the Yoga Sutra: Samadhi Pada

The Practice of the Yoga Sutra: Sadhana Pada

Upcoming Books in This Series

The Power of the Yoga Sutra: Vibhuti Pada

The Promise of the Yoga Sutra: Kaivalya Pada

Also by Pandit Rajmani Tigunait, PhD

Sri Sukta: Tantra of Inner Prosperity

Vishoka Meditation: The Yoga of Inner Radiance

The Pursuit of Power and Freedom: Katha Upanishad

Touched by Fire: The Ongoing Journey of a Spiritual Seeker

Lighting the Flame of Compassion

Inner Quest: Yoga's Answers to Life's Questions

The Himalayan Masters: A Living Tradition

Why We Fight: Practices for Lasting Peace

At the Eleventh Hour: The Biography of Swami Rama

Swami Rama of the Himalayas: His Life and Mission

Tantra Unveiled: Seducing the Forces of Matter and Spirit

Shakti: The Power in Tantra (A Scholarly Approach)

From Death to Birth: Understanding Karma and Reincarnation

The Power of Mantra and the Mystery of Initiation

Shakti Sadhana: Steps to Samadhi

Seven Systems of Indian Philosoph

The Practice *of the* Yoga Sutra

SADHANA PADA

PANDIT RAJMANI TIGUNAIT, PHD

HIMALAYAN INSTITUTE®

HONESDALE, PENNSYLVANIA USA

Himalayan Institute, Honesdale, PA 18431
HimalayanInstitute.org

Printed in the United States of America

23 22 21 2 3 4 5

ISBN-13: 978-0-89389-279-1 (paper)

Cover design by Meera Tigunait

♾ This paper meets the requirements of ANSI/NISO Z39-48-1992 (Permanence of Paper).

Contents

Introduction

We are aspiring beings. The desire to be better, happier, healthier, more beautiful, and more powerful is inherent in all of us. When this desire dims we begin to shrink, and when it dies we are human in name only.

Normally people believe desire is bad, and further, that desire grows as we grow. But the enlightened masters see the force of desire in a different light. According to them, desires have made us what we are today—we grow in response to our growing desires. There are as many desires as there are stars in the sky. Some are negative and others positive. Some feed our subhuman behaviors while others motivate us to identify and embrace the divine self.

Yogis divide the entire range of desires into three categories: *sattvic, rajasic,* and *tamasic*. Sattvic desires are illuminating. They imbue us with enthusiasm, courage, and indomitable will, inspiring us to discover and embrace the purest and most delightful part of ourselves. Sattvic desires are the agents of our continuous transformation. In their presence, we exude self-confidence.

Rajasic desires pump us up with nervous energy, making us scattered, anxious, and full of doubt. Rajasic desires leave us perpetually dissatisfied and impel us to seek and embrace short-lived sensory pleasures. In their presence, we are not happy with what we have and chase what we do not have, only to drop it for something else.

Tamasic desires cast a veil of inertia over our enthusiasm, courage, and willpower. In their presence, we become fatalistic and lethargic—we find it pleasant to sink into a stupor.

The minds of ordinary people are dominated by the interplay of these three categories of desire. We become exceptional when we free our mind from this interplay and train it to embrace only illuminating desires. This training is yoga.

Patanjali's *Yoga Sutra* is the most complete text on the philosophy and practice of yoga. It consists of 196 sutras divided into four chapters: "Samadhi Pada," "Sadhana Pada," "Vibhuti Pada," and "Kaivalya Pada."

Patanjali, one of the greatest yogis of all time, distilled the wisdom and experiences of thousands of masters and compressed them into these 196 sutras. With the passage of time, scholars and practitioners expounded on this text. Among these outstanding commentators, the sage Vyasa has long been recognized as the final authority on the intent and content of the *Yoga Sutra*. Following in the footsteps of the tradition, and in conformity with the promptings of my heart and the practice I adopted in writing *The Secret of the Yoga Sutra: Samadhi Pada*, I have treated Patanjali's *Yoga Sutra* and Vyasa's commentary as one in the pages that follow. As confirmed by my own experience and the experiences of generations of practitioners, when we study and practice what this classic text contains, we gain the same experiences as those who came before us.

As we saw in *The Secret of the Yoga Sutra*, at the outset of "Samadhi Pada," Patanjali shares the ultimate yogic insight: the mind is the greatest of all secrets, and mastering the mind and its roaming tendencies empowers us to attain victory in both our inner and outer worlds. Patanjali considers yoga and *samadhi*, the absolutely peaceful and inwardly focused mind, to be synonymous. In "Samadhi Pada," he delineates a plan that we can adopt to train our mind and free it from its self-defeating habits. He tells us that a disturbed and confused mind cannot lead us to victory in either the worldly or spiritual realms. Only after we have acquired a clear, calm, perceptive, and discerning mind are we able to differentiate essentials from non-essentials and set a goal for achieving lasting happiness. In the first chapter, Patanjali emphasizes the need for purifying our mind and turning it inward, where it has the opportunity to bathe in the luminosity of the divine being. This is enlightenment. An enlightened mind is free from all fear and doubt. It neither grieves over the past nor is anxious about the future. It stands still, enjoying its union with the divine. This is samadhi.

"Samadhi Pada" is written for those who aspire to nothing short of samadhi. It is for those who know that life is much too precious to be consumed by the charms and temptations of the world. However, the second chapter, "Sadhana Pada," is for those of us caught in the day-to-day struggles of life. For most of us, samadhi is a far-fetched dream. We are so consumed by the reality of pain, sorrow, fear, and grief that the urgency to overcome it supersedes all spiritual pursuits. This chapter, then, is for most of us.

Here, in "Sadhana Pada," Patanjali describes a systematic approach to yoga practice. It begins with the acknowledgement of a harsh reality—pain—and goes on to remind us how entrenched we have become in the habit of denying that we are in pain until we are engulfed by it. Ours is a culture that views pain as a physical condition and encourages us to cure it by swallowing a pill. Even though most of us know pain also has a deeper, emotional dimension, we fail to recognize that treating sorrow and emotional torment is as urgent as treating physical pain. We shy away from exploring the deeper dimension of pain and its crippling effect on life as a whole. Yet this exploration is precisely what is required if we are to live the life of freedom and joy to which all of us aspire.

The Sanskrit word for pain and sorrow is *duhkha*. This broad term includes the most familiar forms of physical pain as well as fear, grief, depression, dementia, and every other condition that causes us to experience life as burdensome. Pain in any form drains the vitality of our body and mind. It disconnects us from our innate sense of beauty and goodness and hampers our ability to enjoy what we have and what we are.

In "Sadhana Pada," Patanjali charts a succinct and straightforward plan to transcend pain and embrace lasting happiness. He divides his plan into four parts: acknowledge the dynamics of pain (*heya*); discover the root cause of pain (*heya-hetu*); identify the state in which there is no pain (*hana*); and apply the tools to reach that state (*hana-upaya*).

In the process of explaining the pervasive nature of pain and sorrow, Patanjali demonstrates that disease and old age do not walk into our lives alone. They are always accompanied by carelessness, denial, attachment, and unbending likes and dislikes. This battalion of inner enemies creates an environment of confusion, fear, and doubt, which quickly becomes a breeding ground for anger, hatred, jealousy, and greed. These enemies damage our power of discernment. Our clarity of mind plummets. Our mental faculties become so dull they no longer efficiently guide and govern the systems of our body. This is how the subtle dynamism of pain upsets the internal ecology of our body and mind, setting the stage for disease and old age.

To show the root cause of pain, Patanjali takes us to a realm too subtle to be easily comprehensible—the karmic impressions stored in our mind. Patanjali calls these karmic impressions "afflictions." He divides all afflictions into five broad categories: our unwillingness to examine the validity of what we believe to be true (*avidya*); unwavering faith in our distorted self-identity (*asmita*); attachment to what appears to be us and ours (*raga*); aversion to what poses a threat to what we are and what we own (*dvesha*); and fear of losing ourselves and our familiar world (*abhinivesha*). These afflictions have become a living part of us. From deep within, they influence our thoughts and feelings, which in turn influence every part of our body as well as our mind. Our actions are outward expressions of our thoughts and feelings. Patanjali details how the afflictions propel our actions, how our actions in turn strengthen the afflictions, and finally, how our actions and afflictions work together to perpetuate our pain and sorrow.

Next Patanjali reminds us of the truth grounded in his personal experience and in the experiences of a long line of masters: we are pure beings, and as such we transcend even the subtlest trace of pain and sorrow. Discovering our pure being is our birthright. There is no higher achievement than discovering our pure self and no greater loss than dying without knowing who we are. When we discover our pure self we become aware of life's purpose. This fills us with newfound vigor, vitality, enthusiasm, and the conviction that finding life's purpose is our destiny. This conviction frees us from attachment to the past and uncertainty about the future. This is freedom—the ground for lasting happiness.

Finally, Patanjali provides a systematic practice for reaching this lofty goal. Before unveiling this practice, he reminds us of our relationship with our creator, our place in the world, and the role of worldly resources and experiences in enabling us to find life's purpose. As he explains, the world evolves from *prakriti*, primordial nature. Prakriti is the intrinsic power of the absolute divine being. Every aspect of creation is infused with the power of primordial nature. Our body, mind, and senses are the tools for discovering nature's bounty as well as the repository of nature's infinite riches. The systematic practice of yoga enables us to access nature's treasury within us and outside us. It is in this context that Patanjali presents the practice of yoga in eight parts (*ashtanga yoga*).

The first two parts, the *yamas* and *niyamas*, are contemplative tools for living a healthy and peaceful life. They enable us to build a world free from violence, dishonesty, greed, addiction, and possessiveness. While living in this unique world, we are not a threat to others and others are not a threat to us. Patanjali helps us explore all the obstacles—known and unknown—that may prevent us from creating this ideal world, and delineates a clear plan for removing them.

The remaining six parts of ashtanga yoga focus on the techniques for mastering our body, mind, and senses. Like steps in a ladder, each part serves as the foundation for the next. *Asana*, the third part, enables us to master our body and reclaim its natural strength, stamina, and flexibility. When practiced with focus and precision, asana restores our innate beauty, charm, vigor, and self-healing power. This forms the ground for the fourth step, *pranayama*. Pranayama enables us to access the immense pool of *prana*, the life force that links and sustains the body and mind. Awakened by the practice of pranayama, the life force empowers the body and mind to enhance their mutually supportive relationship. The mind becomes acutely aware of the body's needs and comes forward to meet them. The body senses the mind's intent and responds spontaneously.

The remaining four parts of yoga practice unfold from here. This entire sequence—collecting the scattered forces of the mind (*pratyahara*), bringing them to their home base (*dharana*), turning the mind inward to discover its immense powers and privileges (*dhyana*), and finally, bringing all of our mental powers to bear on discovering and uniting ourselves with our pure being (*samadhi*)—is a natural process of spiritual unfoldment, provided we practice the first four steps of yoga perfectly and precisely.

Patanjali reminds us that perfection and precision in the practice of yoga come from *tapas*, *svadhyaya*, and *Ishvara pranidhana*. *Tapas* means "austerity"; *svadhyaya*, "self-study"; and *Ishvara pranidhana*, "trustful surrender to higher reality." These three together constitute *kriya yoga*, the force that brings the practice of yoga to life. Yoga sadhana leads to self-mastery only in conjunction with these three factors. Without them, yoga is merely a skill.

The yogic approach to practicing tapas is completely different from what we commonly think of as austerity. Tapas is a precise, regimented set of disciplines that enable us to awaken the inherent power of our body and mind and then use that power to overcome our inertia, sloth, and carelessness.

Similarly, svadhyaya, or self-study, entails more than simply reflecting on the current condition of our mind. It is an extremely refined practice that connects us to our own inner brilliance—the shining being within us. Once connected to this inner brilliance, we are free from all fears and doubts and are thus empowered to do our practice wholeheartedly.

In the same way, the third component, Ishvara pranidhana, is more than merely believing in God. Trustful surrender to higher reality is a well-defined practice that leads to experiencing the presence of higher reality in every breath we take. It is a practice that engenders a constant awareness of our creator, guide, and provider. This awareness removes even the slightest possibility of self-isolation and self-alienation. It frees us from the subtlest pain of all—loneliness.

When even one of these eight limbs of yoga—asana, for example—is practiced in the light of tapas, svadhyaya, and Ishvara pranidhana, it will open the door to infinite possibilities. When all eight of them are practiced methodically in this light, the promise of yoga is fulfilled: we are the highest expression of our creator's joy and we are destined to experience that joy. That is the subject of this volume.

SADHANA PADA

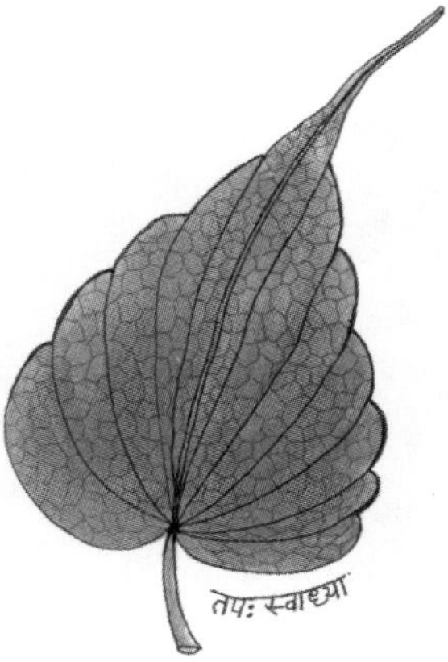

SUTRA 2:1

तपःस्वाध्यायेश्वरप्रणिधानानि क्रियायोगः ॥१॥

tapaḥsvādhyāyeśvarapraṇidhānāni kriyāyogaḥ ॥ 1 ॥

tapaḥ, austerity or heat; *svādhyāya*, self-study or self-reflection; *īśvarapraṇidhāna*, trustful surrender to Ishvara; *kriyāyogaḥ*, yoga in action

Yoga in action is composed of austerity, self-study, and trustful surrender to Ishvara.

P*rakriti,* primordial nature, is infinitely rich. She is the apex of beauty, joy, and creativity—the ground and source of everything that exists. Prakriti is the culmination of intelligence and ingenuity. Every part of us—body, mind, breath, thought, speech, and action—is infused with the infinite beauty, joy, and creativity of primordial nature. We are the ultimate expression of her intrinsic richness. We are what she is—nothing more and nothing less. In all our endeavors, both conscious and unconscious, we are striving to experience this richness.

As we saw in *The Secret of the Yoga Sutra: Samadhi Pada,* human beings are the finest aspect of creation. Our body and mind serve as a gateway to the boundless beauty, joy, and intelligence that is in us and is us. Yoga is the method we use to discover our inherent wealth, a subject expounded on in detail in the first chapter of the *Yoga Sutra*. There, the core of yoga sadhana is *samadhi,* the sublime state of mental purity and stillness.

Samadhi is the epitome of fulfillment and freedom. We reach it through *abhyasa* and *vairagya. Abhyasa,* normally translated as "practice," requires us to employ our mind to flow peacefully inward for a prolonged period without interruption and with reverence. *Vairagya,* normally translated as "non-attachment," requires us to disassociate our mind from afflicting thoughts. The combined forces of abhyasa and vairagya lead us through different stages of samadhi to a state of *vishoka,* the self-luminous joy that is our core being (YS 1:36).

Vishoka manifests when we apply the techniques of abhyasa and vairagya by meditating on the lotus of our heart. This is a subtle process, one that requires a laser-focused mind. We cultivate this highly focused mind by concentrating on extraordinary sensory objects, which, according to Patanjali, are locked in different niches of our body (YS 1:35). Becoming aware of these extraordinary sensory objects is a great accomplishment. Concentrating and meditating on them requires mastering the art of entering the deeper dimensions of our body and sense organs and capturing sensory experiences from within. This is easy for an accomplished yogi, but for most of us it appears to be so far out of reach that it almost seems like a fantasy.

The techniques of yoga Patanjali described in the first chapter of the *Yoga Sutra,* "Samadhi Pada," are meant for those who have a reasonably one-pointed mind. Such seekers are largely free from disturbing, stupefying, and distracting mental tendencies. They understand they must employ their physical, mental, and spiritual resources to discover their pristine being and become established in it. Comparatively speaking, they are accomplished yogis in search of the tools and means to further accelerate their quest—tools Patanjali provides in "Samadhi Pada."

The second chapter of the *Yoga Sutra*, "Sadhana Pada," begins with the recognition that we have lost much of the innate wisdom of our body and the immense power of our mind—they no longer exude the wisdom and power granted us by nature. We rarely experience the grounding quality of the earth or the freedom of movement inherent in the air. We are more often tired and depleted than vibrant and energetic. At the mental level, we are more prone to doubt, fear, anger, grief, and feelings of powerlessness than we are to clarity, self-confidence, fortitude, happiness, and self-trust. But despite these physical and mental limitations, we are aspiring yogis—we are trying to find life's purpose. The system of yoga practice described here in the second chapter is beneficial for aspiring and accomplished yogis alike. Patanjali calls this system *kriya yoga.*

Kriya yoga is a significant term. *Kriya* means "ability to act, ability to move." Kriya is the dynamic power of action, which moves by its own intrinsic virtue and sets inert matter in motion. This word is more easily understood when juxtaposed with the word *karma*. Although both *kriya* and *karma* can be translated as "action," there is a vast difference between them. Both are derived from the verb root *kri* (*dukṛṅ* in the Paninian system), which means "to do." *Kriya* refers to an action in process as well as to the dynamic force propelling the action. *Karma* refers to a completed action. Unless a fresh wave of action is exerted on karma, it remains unchanged. Karma is an unchanging field of completed action waiting to be harvested by the performer of the action, while kriya is ever-moving, ever-expanding energy. Kriya yoga is yoga *in* action, not the yoga *of* action, and should not be confused with karma yoga.

According to the masters of Sri Vidya, *kriya shakti,* the power of action, is the core of yoga. In the Sri Vidya tradition, the absolute divinity is described as Tripura, the one who pervades, permeates, and transcends the reality corresponding to the states of waking, dreaming, and dreamless sleep. She is composed of three intrinsic attributes: *iccha shakti*, the power of will; *jnana shakti*, the power of knowledge; and *kriya shakti*, the power of action. Will and knowledge exert their force only when animated by the power of action. The power of action shakes off the inertia blanketing our soul. It awakens our dormant forces of will and knowledge and infuses us with self-trust and self-confidence. In the light of this active will and knowledge we are able to see ourselves, discover our own strength, and awaken and deploy our dormant forces. Kriya shakti, our intrinsic power of action, is the hallmark of yoga. In the fifty-five sutras of this chapter, Patanjali describes the nature of kriya shakti and provides the methodology for acquiring it.

Every human is an island of excellence. On the material plane, the human body and mind are the crown of creation. To be born as a human is the finest gift and the greatest opportunity. The power inherent in our body and mind is immense. Nature has provided the tools and means we need to discover this immensity and to find the fulfillment and freedom we are seeking. No achievement is greater than discovering what our body and mind hold, and no loss greater than losing our body and mind without discovering the wealth hidden in them. Our unbridled desire to live a long time (for eternity, we hope) is clear evidence that deep within we know the value of a human birth. We know our body and mind are the repository of priceless gifts and we have been given the tools and means to discover those gifts. Yoga is the means, but it is effective only when it is put into action.

The force that infuses our practice with vibrancy is kriya shakti, which is another term for *yoga shakti*. Without this shakti, our practice is lifeless. Kriya yoga is the practice that empowers us to acquire this shakti. Thus kriya yoga is *shakti sadhana,* a fact Patanjali presents in 4:34, his concluding sutra. Kriya yoga awakens the powers lying dormant in our body and mind.

In sutras 2:43–2:45 and sutras 3:45–3:48, Patanjali asserts that a methodical practice of kriya yoga enables us to acquire *kaya siddhi,* mastery over the powers inherent in our body, and *indriya siddhi,* mastery over the powers inherent in our mind and senses. With this mastery, we reclaim our pristine, powerful body and mind, and so are able to identify obstacles and conquer even those that appear insurmountable. With this kind of body and mind we have the ability to practice what is described in sutras 1:33–1:36; experience *vishoka,* the intrinsic joy unstained by even the subtlest trace of sorrow; and become established in *jyotishmati,* the inner luminosity that is our very core.

The forces that bring yoga to fruition are *tapas, svadhyaya,* and *Ishvara pranidhana.* These three forces are the core of yoga. As we examine the nature of each one, it will become clear why Patanjali gives them so much importance.

The standard translation of *tapas* is "austerity," which has a religious connotation. In most religions, austerity is the hallmark of piety. The practice of austerity is associated with dietary restrictions and disciplines that cause discomfort, such as prolonged fasting; subsisting on a diet excluding grain, dairy, salt, and fried food; taking cold baths; staying awake all night; lying on a bed of nails; and refusing to protect oneself from the elements. Patanjali's system of yoga has no room for such austerities, as we will see when he addresses tapas again in sutras 2:32 and 2:43.

The literal meaning of *tapas* is "heat, radiant fire." Practice that ignites our inner fire, brings out our inner radiance, and makes us vibrant and energetic is tapas. Practice that awakens us from our deep-seated slumber and infuses our mind with the radiance we had before we began our journey into this world is tapas. Practice that enables us to recapture the joy and spontaneity of childhood and the enthusiasm and stamina of youth is tapas. Practice that fills us with vitality and with the enthusiasm and courage to discover the unknown spheres of life is tapas.

To understand why tapas is so powerful, we need to understand how we have drained the inherent power and wisdom from our body and mind. We begin our journey to this world with a clear purpose: lasting fulfillment and ultimate freedom. Before entering the world we had a glimpse of the lord of life, the knower of all the tendencies and subtle impressions stored in our mind (YS 4:18). We experienced his unconditional love and the thrilling realization that he has always been with us. But as soon as we enter the world, we are sucked back into the mental conditions that enveloped our consciousness when we were dying. Old habits formed in previous lives; the powerful urges of fear, hunger, sleep, and self-preservation; the desire to possess and consume; an unwillingness to let go; inferiority and superiority complexes; feelings of incompetence and powerlessness; mistrust in our own judgment; and reliance on the opinions of others all return in full force. With little awareness of what we are doing, we fall back into our prior mental conditioning.

As we grow up, the reality created by this mental conditioning strengthens until it veils our true identity—our pure and pristine self. As a result, our intuition and intelligence are compromised. The mind becomes dull and dense and the body's innate wisdom declines. We become highly susceptible to the conditions imposed by our surroundings and live without giving much thought to what is right and wrong, good and bad, healthy and unhealthy. In other words, our pure and pristine being has been subdued by the world of our mental conditioning. We have lost a substantial part of our perceptive and discerning mind: we confuse sloth with comfort, possession with prestige, consumption with enjoyment, and indulgence with fulfillment. In a climate pervaded by carelessness, we search for freedom.

As the grip of carelessness tightens, we lose sight of the reality regarding ourselves and our inherent power and wisdom. Our senses grab sensory objects indiscriminately. Our perception of pleasure and nourishment becomes distorted. Our tastes and interests are no longer guided by our innate wisdom—we adopt a lifestyle without weighing its merits and demerits. Our sleep and eating habits and our feelings of pleasure and pain are no longer compatible with our inner drive for happiness and nourishment. We have become disconnected from ourselves—our body and mind are no longer in full view of our consciousness. Our knowledge of our body and mind shrinks until we know very little about ourselves. We stumble through life on autopilot. We eat, drink, and sleep. We engage in sensory pleasures. We labor to meet the demands of our body and the world around us. The result? We employ our body and mind under pressure from external forces without clearly understanding the real motives behind our actions. Because this causes enormous wear and tear on both body and mind, healing and nourishing ourselves becomes more important than using our body and mind to find lasting fulfillment and ultimate freedom.

Most of us fail to recognize fatigue and exhaustion as serious conditions with the potential to cripple our innate abilities: our power of discernment, memory, and will; the brain's capacity to regulate our internal organs; and the heart's ability to hear and heed the voice of our soul. We realize we have a problem only when our body is impaired and our mental abilities have declined. Even then we refuse to recognize that these alarming conditions have a deeper cause and look for a quick fix instead. As soon as the condition seems to have abated, we resume our old habits. This has led us to develop a complex disease-management industry, while ignoring the need to acquire a vibrant body and a self-luminous, joyful mind. As a solution to this seemingly intractable problem, Patanjali advises us to embrace tapas.

In practice, tapas means refraining from unwholesome activities and adopting a lifestyle that supports the practice of yoga. The life of a yogi is one of purpose, the first and foremost of which is keeping our most highly prized wealth—our body, mind, and senses—fully protected. Carelessness, sloth, inertia, and unhealthy eating habits are our greatest enemies. These enemies are sneaky—they cast a veil of illusion over our mind, convincing us that they are our best friends. As a result, we run after habits that harm our body, mind, and senses. Withstanding the allure of such habits is tapas.

Because in the beginning, acting against the dictates of these habits seems like torture, tapas is commonly described as austerity. Embracing austerity without right understanding is painful. We embrace tapas joyfully only when we are able to see the immense rewards it brings.

To help us understand the crucial role of tapas in both our daily life and our spiritual quest, Patanjali introduces svadhyaya.

Svadhyaya is a composite of *sva* and *adhyaya. Sva* means "one's own." More precisely, as Patanjali and Vyasa explain in sutra 2:23, *sva* means "the power of one's self; the power of the objective world that we try to own, embrace, and consume." *Adhyaya* means "study, contemplate, examine." Thus *svadhyaya* means "to study, examine, and reflect on ourselves, our internal states, the objects of our senses, and the current condition of our body and mind, as well as on the thoughts, feelings, and opinions that are so dear to us." For the sake of simplicity, we can translate *svadhyaya* as "self-study." Self-study requires that we make an inventory of our physical and mental resources and assess the vitality of our body and the rate at which we are expending it. It also requires that we remain vigilant and avoid dissipating the power of our mind with unwholesome activities.

The job of the senses is to collect experiences and present them to the mind, but it is the mind's job to use those experiences to find lasting fulfillment and ultimate freedom. In an attempt to embrace and assimilate sensory pleasures, we must be careful not to drain the vitality of our body, damage our senses, and dissipate our mental energy. To this end, we must employ *viveka shakti,* the power of discernment, to help us differentiate pleasure from indulgence. From a practical standpoint then, svadhyaya is the process of employing the power of discernment and maintaining a constant awareness of who we are, what we are trying to become, and how the objective world can help us accomplish our goal.

According to Vyasa, we put the principle of self-study into practice by undertaking a well-defined course of *japa,* repetition of sacred sounds and mantras. As described in sutras 1:27 and 1:28, japa enables our mind to travel toward the center of consciousness without being distracted by the charms and temptations of the world. With japa we reach the self-luminous, peaceful space within, but we also become aware of the dark place from where our unwanted agitating thoughts arise. As the power of mantra japa quiets our mind, we are able to see our subtle desires, cravings, and ambitions more vividly. We become aware of the unknown parts of ourselves, including those that are painful and frightening. This provides an opportunity to identify what we must renounce in order to advance in our quest—what we must let go of in order to acquire something new and auspicious.

This is how japa turns into self-study. Our process of self-examination becomes precise. We no longer flounder around with abstract philosophical ideas, such as whether or not our soul is in bondage, whether God is our savior, or whether the objective world is real or illusory. We are acutely aware of the roaming tendencies of our mind and are convinced we must attain freedom from them. We also know which tendencies are most problematic. In the climate of self-examination created by mantra japa we are able to set our priorities. We employ our power of discernment, reflect on the trivial nature of our mental distractions, and remind ourselves that life is too precious to allow it to be consumed by the demands of the world.

The study of scripture is another way of putting the principle of self-study into practice. In ancient India, a text that embodied knowledge capable of guiding and leading us to the highest goal of life was regarded as *shastra,* scripture. The Vedas and the Upanishads were prime examples. However, with the passage of time, numerous other texts, including those expounding on mundane subjects like medicine, ethics, politics, rituals, astrology, and philosophy, began to be treated as scriptures, as did epics about kings and saints. Elaborating on the concept of svadhyaya, Vyasa emphasizes that only those texts that embody indisputable knowledge showing us the path to ultimate freedom are an essential component of self-study. In other words, svadhyaya entails the study of spiritual texts that are authentic, contain experiential knowledge, and are infused with the energy to guide us on the path of inner freedom.

Japa and the study of scripture are complementary practices. For example, during the tranquil moments of absorption in japa, a realization may dawn about the need to change our direction in life. We are thrilled, for we know this change will take us to the highest goal, but we are also frightened, for we know complying with it will require walking away from the cherished world of our desires and ambitions. In such situations, guidance from scriptures grounded in experiential knowledge is extremely helpful. The term for this is *shastra kripa,* grace of scripture. The tradition considers the grace of the scriptures as important as *Ishvara kripa,* grace of God, and *atma kripa,* grace of oneself, which manifests in the form of self-effort.

The third principle that brings our yoga practice to fruition is *Ishvara pranidhana,* trustful surrender to God. In "Samadhi Pada," Patanjali introduced trustful surrender as a means to reach samadhi (YS 1:23–1:29). There he described God as our inner guide, protector, provider, and eternal companion. As soon as we open ourselves to her unconditional love and guidance, the roaming tendencies of our mind subside and we reach the highest level of self-realization, which dawns in samadhi. Opening ourselves to her loving grace is trustful surrender, and japa is the means (YS 1:27–1:28). In "Samadhi Pada," Patanjali makes it clear that surrender to God is a complete path, and he makes this point again in "Sadhana Pada": "From trustful surrender, comes *samadhi siddhi*" (YS 2:45). But here, in sutra 2:1, he introduces trustful surrender as one of the three essential forces that breathe life into our yoga sadhana and ensure that we reach perfection, even though at the outset we do not have a clear, tranquil, one-pointed, spiritually inclined, and discerning mind.

Here Patanjali is not treating Ishvara pranidhana as an independent path of sadhana but rather as a force which, coupled with tapas and svadhyaya, brings our yoga sadhana to fruition. At a practical level, tapas, svadhyaya, and Ishvara pranidhana are inseparable—they breathe life into each other, and together they breathe life into our sadhana. These three forces are essential to all the practices Patanjali introduces throughout the *Yoga Sutra*. But for now we will focus on the application of Ishvara pranidhana in the context of kriya yoga.

As Vyasa explains, offering all our activities into the highest guru (*sarva kriyanam parama-gurau arpanam*) and renouncing the fruits of those activities (*tat-phala-sanyaso va*) are Ishvara pranidhana. To understand what Vyasa means by this statement, we need to analyze the words he uses. In the first part of the statement, "offering all our activities into the highest guru," he uses *kriya* instead of *karma*. He also uses the locative case instead of the accusative case for the term *parama-guru*, highest guru. Furthermore, Vyasa is elaborating on Ishvara pranidhana while using the word *parama-guru* instead of *Ishvara*. A careful analysis of these words will help us arrive at an understanding of Ishvara pranidhana.

The literal meaning of *kriya* is "verb." Every verb is representative of a distinct process or function and no process or function reaches fruition without a doer. The word for "doer" is *karta*. Panini, the predecessor of Patanjali, defines *karta* as *svatantrah karta*, "in regard to performing an action, the one who is self-governed (*svatantra*) is the doer."

In the light of this definition, because our knowledge and capacities are limited, we are not the doer of our actions. The source of our inspiration, motivation, and decisions is too subtle to comprehend. We have little understanding of our own biological functions and no understanding of the subtler forces and causes that trigger a cascade of changes in our mind and consciousness. Our decisions are strongly influenced by emotional impulses. Most of our actions do not have their source in reason, yet we claim to be both the doer and the sole proprietor of those actions. Our problems begin when we identify ourselves as the doer of our actions, forgetting that there is a self-governed intelligent force that has endowed us with the ability to perform actions. We forget that both the fruits of actions and the dynamic that propels the phenomenon we perceive as an action are entirely dependent on higher intelligence. This intelligence is Ishvara (*Bhagavad Gita* 18:61).

An example may be helpful. Take two sentences: Hercules lifts the earth. Einstein solves the mystery of the universe. At a mundane level, Hercules and Einstein are *karta,* the doers, for without them the earth would not have been lifted or the mystery of the universe solved. At another level, however, it is childish to credit Hercules with lifting the earth and Einstein with solving an impenetrable mystery. There is a higher intelligence—the self-governing force—and when that intelligence manifests, we emerge as Hercules and Einstein. Our mind and senses are the instruments of this intelligent force. In other words, although we are instrumental in the performance of an action, the real performer is higher intelligence. Identifying ourselves as the doer of our actions is pure ignorance and leads to bondage. Only when we understand that the higher intelligence in us is the actual doer are we able to surrender the fruits of our actions. Disidentification with our actions empowers us with the wisdom and courage to surrender the fruits of our actions to the real doer.

Vyasa's use of *parama-guru,* the highest teacher, instead of *Ishvara,* is highly significant. He does not want the concept of God—which has become the exclusive domain of theology and is often described in the language of mythology—to contaminate the yogic understanding of higher reality. As we have seen in sutras 1:23–1:29, Ishvara is utterly different from the concept of

God in the various religious traditions. In yoga, God is not an entity separate from us and residing outside us. God is not a person but an ever-present guiding intelligence. It is a reality without a persona. To further emphasize this fact, Vyasa formulates his sentence to mean that Ishvara pranidhana is "offering all of our actions *into* parama-guru" instead of "*to* parama-guru." The way this sentence is constructed makes it clear that parama-guru, the highest teacher, is not an entity consisting of a discrete body to whom we hand over our actions and the fruits of our actions. It is *purusha vishesha,* the unique category of reality (YS 1:24–26), into which we offer our actions and their fruits.

This offering is accompanied by the understanding that we ourselves and the phenomenal world around us are guided by the ever-present inner intelligence. Everything that happens is happening at the will of this unfathomable force. It is a privilege to be instrumental in an action initiated and executed by this force. Therefore, according to Vyasa, Ishvara pranidhana means offering our sense of identification as the doer of our actions into the ever-present guiding intelligence.

Let us examine what happens when we do not acknowledge our instrumentality and instead cling to the belief that we are the doers of the actions we perform.

At this stage in our evolution, the capacity of our body has diminished and the clarity of our mind is compromised. For the most part, our actions are governed by our habits. Our desires, ambitions, and decisions are shaped by our likes and dislikes. Our understanding of good and bad, right and wrong, is stained by doubt, fear, anger, hatred, jealousy, and self-importance. In this mental environment, our actions are inevitably contaminated. Actions create impressions in the mind, further distorting our understanding. This is the law of karma. As this cycle continues, we become less and less aware of the reality pertaining to ourselves and our relationship with the objective world. If this cycle is not checked, we become the product of our own distorted understanding, which yogis call *avidya.* Karmic impressions are as real to the children of avidya as samadhi is to the yogis.

Karmic impressions—*samskaras*—are the building blocks of our mental world. They are hard to renounce. We have earned them by investing our most prized wealth, our sense of doership. Every action and its results carry the fingerprints of our doership. The impressions created by our actions retain the qualities and attributes of our actions. Karmic impressions form the content of our mind—they are firmly established in us. Our samskaras are our possessions; our bond with them is ancient and grows stronger every day. Our samskaras have molded us into what we have become today—they shape our reality. In short, they are us and we are them. Our bond with them is so strong that losing them feels like losing ourselves. That is why even though our karmic impressions are inevitably accompanied by fear and pain, letting go of them is difficult.

The dearer an object, the more we fear losing it. An object is dear because we have invested our most valued wealth—our sense of doership—in it. When we lose a child, a spouse, power, or money, we experience pain in proportion to our identification with ourselves as parents, soul mates, or magnates. We do not like pain, yet we do not know how to let it go. This condition of helplessness forces us to find a justification for our pain. We try to hold someone or something—including God, karma, or destiny—responsible for our suffering. When the pain still does not go away, we become angry. Anger leads to confusion; confusion to delusion; and delusion to loss of memory, linear thinking, and the power of discernment. This accelerating cycle of pain further damages our mental world. Ishvara pranidhana, trustful surrender to God, reverses this cycle and helps us restore our pure and pristine mind.

When put into practice, Ishvara pranidhana is an amazing force. It demolishes the fundamental premise we use to justify our pain. It takes away our justification for crying and complaining. Ishvara pranidhana makes us aware that we have received far more than we have lost. Our reasons to be grateful for what divine providence has given to us supersede any reason for sorrow and grief. The more tightly we embrace the practice of Ishvara pranidhana, the more clearly we see how little we know about the source and nature of consciousness. This realization makes us wiser. It becomes easier for us to detach ourselves from painful thoughts and feelings without losing our sensitivity to conditions that are both real and significant on the material plane. Ishvara pranidhana enables us to operate on two levels simultaneously—spiritual and mundane. We are fully aware of the inner reality and respectful of the forces that dominate our worldly existence. We become citizens of both worlds and have the wisdom to obey and honor the laws of both. We are able to perform our actions skillfully, wisely, and lovingly, and our actions are no longer binding.

Patanjali places so much emphasis on tapas, svadhyaya, and Ishvara pranidhana because they are the core of yoga. In combination, they enable us to reclaim the innate wisdom and power of our body and the self-luminous joy of our mind. A healthy body and a pure mind are essential to any practice.

By applying the principle of tapas as described in the yoga tradition—*yatha-yogam* (Vyasa on YS 2:32)—we detoxify our body, restore its natural balance, awaken its innate intelligence, and fill our limbs and organs with renewed vitality, strength, and energy.

This is what ayurvedic practitioners, tantric alchemists, and Sri Vidya adepts call *kaya kalpa,* total renewal. With tapas, we make the body a perfect conduit for our mind.

Svadhyaya helps us employ the resources of our body and mind for higher achievement. The principal component of svadhyaya is silently repeating sacred mantric sounds, thus training our mind to become quiet and flow inward. This inwardly flowing mind is further employed to examine our internal states and reflect on whether or not we are performing our actions purposefully.

Ishvara pranidhana is a guiding and nurturing force. While anchored in Ishvara pranidhana we are able to withstand and eventually conquer even our greatest fear—the fear of losing ourselves, our loved ones, and our most cherished possessions, our karmic impressions. Together, tapas, svadhyaya, and Ishvara pranidhana are the force behind *kriya,* action, and without kriya there is no yoga.

How action-driven yoga helps us organize our mind, overcome resistance to change, cultivate a taste for higher good, rediscover our self-luminous joyful mind, and become fully established in our essential nature—the reality that is in us and *is* us—is the subject of the next sutra and those that follow.

SUTRA 2:2

समाधिभावनार्थः क्लेशतनूकरणार्थश्च ॥२॥

samādhibhāvanārthaḥ kleśatanūkaraṇārthaśca ॥ 2 ॥

samādhi, a completely still state of mind; the highest state of spiritual absorption; *bhāvana*, to induce; *arthaḥ*, objective; *kleśa*, affliction; *tanūkaraṇa*, the process of eliminating or minimizing; *artha*, objective; *ca*, and

The objective of yoga is to induce samadhi and attenuate the afflictions.

In "Samadhi Pada," Patanjali defines yoga as mastery over the roaming tendencies of the mind (YS 1:2). Here he tells us that when put into practice, yoga leads to samadhi and attenuates the *kleshas,* the afflictions that are the subtlest cause of sorrow. Samadhi is a perfectly still, pristine state of mind. In samadhi we gain the direct experience of our essential nature and become aware of the fullness of our being. We are free from the mental conditioning of our mind—there are no boundaries around our consciousness. In this consummate state, we experience our oneness with the highest divinity, Ishvara. In samadhi, the purity of our mind is equal to the purity of Ishvara (YS 3:55). Reaching samadhi is a rare opportunity. It requires effort, and to be effective that effort must be methodical.

As we saw in "Samadhi Pada," there are various states of samadhi. They can be divided into two parts: higher and lower.

Higher samadhi is the pinnacle of our quest, the state in which we experience our oneness with the highest divinity. Because no cognitions and notions pertaining to our individuality remain, this state of realization is called *asamprajnata samadhi,* samadhi without cognition. All cognitions—all fragments of awareness—have dissolved into pure consciousness (YS 1:18).

Lower samadhi has four distinct stages (YS 1:17). In the first stage, our mind is free from disturbances, stupefaction, and distractions, but still occupied by the gross form of the object of meditation. In the second stage, the mind rises above the gross form of the object and retains only the subtle form. In the third stage, the mind rises above both the gross and subtle forms of the meditative object and is absorbed in the joy induced by meditation itself. In the fourth stage, the mind has transcended both the gross and subtle forms of the object and is absorbed in the pure sense of I-am-ness.

The difference between the third and fourth stages is characterized by the meditative feeling that serves as a gateway to mental absorption. Both the third and fourth stages are extremely refined experiences of samadhi (YS 1:42–46). Beyond this lies the highest state of samadhi, where the yogi's awareness of the object of meditation, the process of meditation, and himself as a meditator have become indistinguishable. In this sublime state, all subtle impressions have been purified and absorbed into the infinitely vast and pristine mental field. All the causes of affliction have been attenuated; there is no possibility of any inner or outer unrest (YS 1:51). Between the lower stages of samadhi and the highest stage, Patanjali describes a transitional stage known as *dharma megha samadhi* (YS 1:47–50, 3:48–53, 4:30–32).

At the practical level, the lower and higher states of samadhi are a continuum. Higher samadhi is the destination of our inner quest, and lower samadhi is the process leading to that destination. Each of us has our own starting point, and we must proceed at our own pace. The starting point is determined by our physical and mental capacities, but the pace of the journey is determined by how easily we are able to overcome the obstacles we encounter.

In "Samadhi Pada," Patanjali delineates nine obstacles and five offshoots (YS 1:30–31) and provides a solution for overcoming them (YS 1:32). But that solution is available only to those who have already arrested the mind's roaming tendencies. It applies only to those who have risen above disturbed, stupefied, and distracted mental states and have cultivated a one-pointed, still, and peaceful mind. In "Samadhi Pada," Patanjali is addressing aspirants with an intense desire to reach samadhi—seekers who are endowed with faith, vigor, retentive power, stillness of mind, and intuitive wisdom (YS 1:20). Even when such seekers encounter obstacles, they are able to focus their mind on a single reality, Ishvara (YS 1:32).

But here, in "Sadhana Pada," Patanjali is offering those of us whose minds are not yet still and one-pointed a means of overcoming obstacles. It is for those whose willpower and determination are relatively weak and whose faith, vigor, retentive power, stillness of mind, and intuitive wisdom are compromised. The practice of yoga described in this chapter leads to samadhi by attenuating the kleshas, afflictions, that are the primary cause of the obstacles and the pain and sorrow they engender.

The most powerful form of misery is *shoka,* sorrow and grief infused with worry, fear, and a sense of powerlessness. By the time we reach this state of misery, we have damaged our rational mind. We are lost, empty, and overcome by hopelessness. This state of mind is sustained by our strong identification with worldly objects and relationships. We are convinced worldly objects and our relationship with them are real and we are incomplete without them; when they prove ephemeral, we are devastated. This sense of devastation contains the seeds of sorrow and grief. As this devastating experience repeats itself, the weight of shoka on our mind and heart becomes heavier. Yet we still continue to insist that the objects of the world and our relationship with them are real. Our unwillingness to examine the validity of this conviction is what yoga calls *avidya*, the ground of all afflictions. All forms of pain and sorrow have their source in this fundamental affliction and are sustained by it.

The ultimate remedy lies in understanding the dynamics of the afflictions and eliminating them once and for all. The next thirteen sutras elaborate on the nature of the afflictions, how they pulsate deep in our mind, and how this pulsation facilitates the relationship between cause and effect, thereby setting the stage for our past actions to bear fruit.

SUTRA 2:3

अविद्यास्मितारागद्वेषाभिनिवेशाः क्लेशाः ॥३॥

avidyāsmitārāgadveṣābhiniveśāḥ kleśāḥ ॥ 3 ॥

avidyā, ignorance; *asmitā*, false sense of self-identity; *rāga*, attachment; *dveṣa*, aversion; *abhiniveśāḥ*, fear of death; *kleśāḥ*, afflictions

Ignorance, false sense of self-identity, attachment, aversion, and fear of death are the afflictions.

The five afflictions—ignorance, false sense of self-identity, attachment, aversion, and fear of death—are the ultimate source of our sorrow. All five are well established in our mind. As long as we are in their grip we will inevitably experience one or more of the nine obstacles: disease, mental inertia, doubt, carelessness, sloth, inability to withdraw from sense cravings, clinging to misunderstanding, inability to reach samadhi, and inability to retain samadhi (YS 1:30). These obstacles breed pain, mental agitation, unsteadiness in our limbs and organs, and disturbances in our inhalation and exhalation (YS 1:31). The nine obstacles and five debilitating conditions accompanying them engulf us in *shoka*, sorrow and grief saturated with worry, fear, and a sense of powerlessness. The entire range of sorrow—from disease to a crippling sense of powerlessness—originates in the *kleshas*, the five afflictions, and is sustained by them.

The subtlest and the most potent affliction is *avidya*, ignorance. We know nothing about the intelligence that constitutes our core being, yet we identify ourselves as the proprietor of intelligence—that is avidya. Our unwillingness to explore ourselves as a force of intelligence, and our strong desire to maintain our ownership of that intelligence, is avidya. From time immemorial we have been nurturing the samskara of our unwillingness to discover our true identity and striving to preserve the identity we believe to be true. Avidya is the subtlest and most deeply seated of all our mental impressions—no other samskara is as strong. *Asmita,* the discrete sense of I-am-ness; *raga,* attachment to that which pleases us; *dvesha,* aversion to that which displeases us; and *abhinivesha,* the fear of losing our possessions—most importantly, our self-identity—are all extensions of avidya.

We are made of the basic constituents of primordial nature—*sattva, rajas,* and *tamas.* These are the *gunas,* the fundamental principles of light, movement, and inertia, respectively. Their mutually supportive functions have made us what we are today (*Sankhya Karika* 13). Sattva keeps the higher purpose of life in full view of our consciousness. Because of sattva, we are intuitive, perceptive, and discerning. Rajas feeds our attachment to worldly objects—we want to possess and consume. Because of rajas, we are ambitious and active. Tamas makes us slothful, uninspired, and fatalistic. Because of tamas, we feel dull and confused.

The awakening of these five afflictions brings a fourfold result: it accelerates the powers of the three gunas—sattva, rajas, and tamas; it lays the foundation for change; it connects the currents of cause and effect; and it brings our actions to fruition (Vyasa on 2:3).

Which guna will be energized when the afflictions awaken, and to what degree, depends on the nature of our afflictions. In other words, our afflictions stir the basic constituents of our mind, awakening some desires and repressing others.

As soon as our afflictions stir the basic constituents of our mind, an atmosphere of excitement is created. We are filled with a desire either to take an action or to refrain from it. We are aware of our intention. We make a decision and that decision is in conformity with our afflictions.

In response to our intention and the willpower invested in materializing it, the forces of cause and effect begin to connect. The intelligence that pervades every nook and cranny of our mind connects the chain of cause and effect and arranges it in proper sequence, thus setting the stage for our previous actions to bear fruit.

The process of deciding to achieve our goal and gathering the forces of our will and determination to materialize what we have decided to achieve is extremely subtle. As we have seen, avidya is our subtlest and most potent samskara. Once it is stirred, the three forces of nature—sattva, rajas, and tamas—are awakened. This awakening lays the foundation for change in both the inner and outer worlds. The subtle forces of our mind and senses and the *tanmatras*, the essential properties of matter, automatically begin to arrange the chain of cause and effect in the proper sequence.

At this stage, the samskaras relevant to achieving our goal have become fully active. Under the influence of these fully awakened and active samskaras, we are determined to achieve our goal and are convinced of the urgency. The samskaras that make this goal so urgent and compelling have momentarily suppressed other samskaras that could have made us doubt the urgency of this goal. Our actions are fully aligned with our samskaras, and in response, all our faculties—ego, intellect, senses, brain, and nervous system—are suffused with the power of action. We employ all our resources to succeed.

Now all five afflictions are working in concert. Ignorance, the false sense of self-identity, attachment, aversion, and fear begin feeding each other and consuming us. At this point our *karma vipaka,* karmic fruition, emerges. Because the process of karmic fruition is extremely subtle, we call it destiny, but destiny is actually the creation of our mind working under the influence of the afflictions. The afflictions themselves are the creation of the mind. Even though it is painful at the core, our attachment to those afflictions is as strong as a stingy person's attachment to his wealth.

If the five afflictions are so well established in each of our minds, why do they not equally affect all of us? Furthermore, why at various times and places are we more affected by one affliction than another? Patanjali answers this question in the next sutra.

SUTRA 2:4

अविद्या क्षेत्रमुत्तरेषां
प्रसुप्ततनुविच्छिन्नोदाराणाम् ॥४॥

avidyā kṣetramuttareṣām
prasuptatanuvicchinnodārāṇām ॥ 4 ॥

avidyā, ignorance; false understanding; *kṣetram*, field; *uttareṣām*, in regard to upcoming ones; *prasupta*, dormant; *tanu*, attenuated; *vicchinna*, disjointed; *udārāṇām*, in regard to those that are already active

Ignorance is the ground for the remaining afflictions, whether they are dormant, attenuated, disjointed, or active.

Ignorance, false sense of self-identity, attachment, aversion, and fear afflict us with sorrow and pain. *Avidya*—ignorance—is the breeding ground for the other four afflictions. Simply put, avidya is our unfamiliarity with ourselves. The deepest groove in our mind is our lack of awareness of who and what we are. Our mind is fully colored by the deep impression of our unawareness of our true identity—we are accustomed to seeing ourselves through this lens. This lack of self-awareness is avidya.

Rooted deeply in our mind, avidya negates our awareness of who we truly are while making us believe we are the owners of our body, mind, and senses, as well as of what we hear, touch, see, taste, and smell. As this avidya-driven belief becomes firmly established, we identify with our body, mind, and senses and with sensory objects. This false sense of self-identity is *asmita*. The difference between avidya and asmita is subtle. In tandem, they claim to be *atman,* the soul. This is the beginning of bondage.

The grip of bondage tightens when *raga*, attachment, *dvesha*, aversion, and *abhinivesha*, fear of death, join avidya and asmita. Our expansive quality shrinks, our comprehension becomes clouded, and our power of discernment plummets. Our priority becomes complying with the cravings of our body, mind, and senses. Life begins to revolve around what we fear most. We become so preoccupied with the chain of pleasant and unpleasant events that we have no energy to conceive of a reality beyond our day-to-day existence. The world of success and failure, loss and gain, honor and insult, fame and humiliation is now our only reality. Blinded by the mysterious forces of avidya and the other four afflictions, we grope our way through life, hoping to find lasting fulfillment and ultimate freedom. This journey leads us nowhere.

The afflictions exist in four different states: *prasupta*, dormant, *tanu*, attenuated, *vicchinna,* disjointed, and *udara,* fully active. Vyasa elaborates on these four states within the context of yoga sadhana and demonstrates how they correspond to different levels of yogic achievement.

In the case of yogis who have achieved *viveka khyati,* intuitive knowledge characterized by clear understanding, the afflictions are *prasupta,* dormant. Like roasted seeds, they have no power to germinate. These yogis have reached *dharma megha samadhi* and beyond (YS 1:50–51). In these higher states of samadhi, the afflictions have been rendered so inert they no longer have the capacity to perform the four functions Vyasa describes in the previous sutra: accelerating the powers of sattva, rajas, and tamas; laying the foundation for change; connecting the current of cause and effect; and bringing our actions to fruition. For all intents and purposes, the afflictions are dead.

Afflictions are *tanu,* attenuated, in those who are actively engaged in yoga sadhana and have wholeheartedly applied the principle of *pratipaksha bhavana,* replacing afflicting thoughts and feelings with those of an opposite nature (YS 2:33). In their case, the afflictions are so weak that even in the presence of circumstances conducive to their awakening, they remain inactive. A yogi whose afflictions are attenuated can clearly see their presence in their subtle form in her mind. She can also see that they have the potential to induce the mind and senses to conform to their demands. But through sadhana, the yogi has developed the capacity to subdue these attenuated afflictions and prevent them from influencing her mind and senses.

Afflictions are *vicchinna,* disjointed, in those who have momentarily subdued some of the afflictions through their yoga sadhana. The other afflictions and the mental turmoil and physical conditions they engender remain fully active. In fact, the dominance of a fully active affliction gives the appearance that the others are weak or dormant. For example, the dominance of anger may give the impression that the seeker is free from afflictions that cause depression or hopelessness. Similarly, in the presence of aversion, attachment seems to be absent. In short, the afflictions that seem to have disappeared are simply waiting their turn to manifest.

Afflictions are *udara,* fully active, in the case of those just beginning their yoga sadhana. These seekers know they have a disturbed, scattered, and confused mind. They know they are suffering from inertia, laziness, and procrastination. They are making an effort to subdue their disturbed, stupefied, distracted mind in favor of a mind that is clear, calm, and focused. They are sincerely trying to adopt a healthy and spiritually rewarding yogic lifestyle. And yet as soon as external circumstances trigger one of the afflictions, they fall from the path of their yoga sadhana. They are easily agitated because they are not yet strong enough to withstand the force of the afflictions. Seekers with fully active afflictions need willpower, determination, tapas, svadhyaya, Ishvara pranidhana, and a custom-designed practice. As we saw in sutra 2:1, this is what Patanjali calls *kriya yoga,* a method of practice that gradually attenuates the afflictions and helps us reach samadhi.

By describing the four states of affliction, Patanjali is addressing the pain and sorrow of all human beings, whether or not they have heard of yoga or regard themselves as yoga practitioners. We are all striving to achieve happiness. Here Patanjali helps each of us assess where we stand in our quest for fulfillment and freedom—and what we must do to reach our goal.

In order to understand how the various states of affliction apply to everyone, it is helpful to examine them in reverse order. Patanjali lists them from top down—dormant to fully active—an order applicable to those familiar with the philosophy and metaphysics of yoga and who aspire to nothing less than samadhi. But when we study these states from bottom up—from fully active to disjointed, attenuated, and finally completely dormant—we can see their practical application in day-to-day life.

Most of us are deeply entrenched in the state in which the afflictions are fully active (*udara*). For example, when we are caught in a particular train of thought and cannot extricate ourselves, we are in the grip of attachment, aversion, and fear. When anger lingers on and on and we are unable to let it go and forgive, we are suffering from asmita, a deep and distorted sense of self-identity. Similarly, prolonged depression, grief, sadness, and hopelessness are rooted in one or more of the afflictions and supported by the others. Our inability to rise above these mental conditions is a sure sign that the afflictions causing them are quite active. This is the situation most of us find ourselves in—we are trying to live a healthy, happy, and peaceful life in a disturbing mental environment.

Deep down we know life is precious and we must not waste it. We know our mind and body are our most precious wealth. We also know we have the tools and means for acquiring perfect health and a joyful mind. This realization may be thickly veiled, but it remains ever present. That is why we aspire to achieve better health, greater wealth, more peace and happiness. In the midst of fully active afflictions—which are stirring the currents of fear, doubt, attachment, desire, aversion, anger, grief, and guilt—we are trying to find lasting fulfillment and freedom. At some point, we realize that if we are to succeed, we must acquire a clear, calm, and one-pointed mind. When this realization dawns, we make an effort to cultivate a one-pointed, peaceful mind. This effort itself is yoga.

As we try to acquire a clear, peaceful, focused mind, our innate wisdom guides us to organize our thought processes, regulate our urges, and discipline our speech and action. Patanjali calls this *tapas*. As soon as the principle of tapas walks into our life, we become more perceptive. We gain enough clarity to reflect on the precious nature of human life and the value of investing life's resources for higher fulfillment. Patanjali calls this *svadhyaya*, self-study. With self-study, we become aware of our inner strengths and weaknesses and the special privileges that come with a human body and mind. We also recognize the power of samskaras, which are constantly feeding our cravings, urges, and habits. These and other insights engendered by self-study fill us with a deep respect for ourselves and the higher divinity, which has always guided, protected, and nurtured us. This is what Patanjali calls *Ishvara pranidhana*, trustful surrender. The quest for higher good through the practice of tapas, svadhyaya, and Ishvara pranidhana is kriya yoga, the surest means of shattering our long-cherished afflictions. As we practice kriya yoga, our fully active afflictions gradually become disjointed (*vicchinna*).

Afflictions that are disjointed lose their strength and do not consume our mind as intensely as when they were fully active. Now we are able to remain quiet and focused—at least for short periods. For example, when we are praying or meditating, we think less frequently about checking our text messages. Thoughts of those we love or hate appear in our mind less often. Then, as the clarity and one-pointedness of our mind increase, we are able to focus longer. We manage our fears and worries more wisely. Because the afflictions that fill our mind with doubt and discourage us from exploring the reality outside the box of our current belief system have become fragmented, we are able to comprehend a previously unknown level of reality. To a great extent, our inner intelligence has escaped the grinding effects of our afflictions.

We know we are on the path of freedom now and we begin to pour our whole heart into our quest. We become more sincere and disciplined. Purifying our mind and making it one-pointed and intuitive no longer feels like work, for we are propelled by inner joy. We begin receiving guidance from the innate wisdom of our body and mind. We know it is important to adopt a life of non-violence, truthfulness, non-possessiveness, cleanliness, contentment, and self-discipline. Laziness is no longer attractive. The internal ecology of our body begins to demand that we revitalize our limbs and organs and stop draining the vitality of our senses. We become acutely aware of the healing power of our breath. In this way, the practices of *asana,* physical exercises, *pranayama,* breathing techniques, and *pratyahara,* withdrawing the senses, evolve naturally. As these practices further purify and nourish our mind, the grip of afflictions weakens and they become attenuated (*tanu*).

This is the most important milestone in our quest, for we are now aware of our central weakness. When the afflictions are attenuated, our mind is clear and steady. We are no longer subject to mood swings. When we feel angry or sad, for example, we know the causes are inside us and so are able to defuse these negative emotions. We are able to reflect on our negative and painful emotions and realize we must replace afflicting thoughts and feelings with non-afflicting ones. We understand we cannot attain freedom from afflicting thoughts simply by ignoring them—the cure lies in identifying the exact nature of the afflicting thought that occupies our mind the most frequently and powerfully and replacing it with its opposite. Patanjali calls this process *pratipaksha bhavana* (YS 2:33).

Pratipaksha bhavana, replacing afflicting thoughts and feelings with those of an opposite nature, requires extraordinary vigilance, courage, and a commitment to eradicating the affliction that serves as a trigger point for all the others. This enables us to withstand the inner unrest caused by the most potent affliction or group of afflictions. They still exist in our mind in subtle form, but due to our high degree of vigilance, courage, and commitment to our practice, these afflictions no longer affect us—the constant awareness of the higher goal of life nullifies their effects and we remain resolute. We continue on the path without becoming sidetracked or distracted. This eventually renders afflictions dormant (*prasupta*). In their dormant state, afflictions have lost their potency and cannot engender mental tendencies. For all intents and purposes, they are dead. Because they have no capacity to feed our samskaras, the mind is free of its roaming tendencies and is at peace. Our vision is no longer clouded—we see the reality pertaining to ourselves, the reality pertaining to our relationship with the divine within, and the reality pertaining to our relationship with the objective world. We are so certain about the truth that questions such as Who am I? Who was I? How and what am I going to be? have vanished (Vyasa on YS 4:25). The *Yoga Sutra* describes this level of mental clarity and inner establishment with terms such as *viveka khyati* (YS 2:26), *taraka* (YS 3:54), *dharma megha* (YS 4:29), *kaivalya, svarupa pratishtha,* and *chiti shakti* (YS 4:34). This level of freedom is the domain of the high-caliber yogis in the category of *videha* and *prakritilaya* (YS 1:19).

According to Vyasa, in these high-caliber masters the fivefold affliction is transformed into *shakti matra,* sheer power. This power contains the essence of the world once run and nurtured by avidya and her four evolutes. Before this transformation, avidya was blocking our vision of reality. It was serving as *ashakti,* the force behind our disempowerment (*Sankhya Karika* 49). This ashakti was damaging our *buddhi sattva,* the essence of our intelligence. Now avidya has turned into *shakti,* the seeing power of the seer. In other words, avidya has been transformed into vidya. The force that once veiled reality has become the conduit for revelation. As we will see in the commentary on sutra 2:20, Vyasa calls this transformed force *jnana vritti,* the mind's self-revealing function.

In the Sri Vidya tradition, this self-revealing force is known as *shuddha vidya,* and the yogi endowed with this power is called *divya augha,* a soul immersed in the stream of divine wisdom. While describing the spiritual nature of such yogis, scriptures say that the divya augha yogis are neither similar to nor dissimilar from the absolute—they are neither one with the absolute nor separate from it. They are neither one nor many. They are beyond duality and non-duality. They have a mind and yet they have no mind. They have samskaras and yet have no samskaras. In the worldly sense, they exist and yet do not exist. In the Sri Vidya tradition, such souls are ranked even above the *siddha* yogis and far above the yogis still confined to their mortal bodies. In our tradition, these high-caliber masters are given five names: *sadyojata, vamadeva, aghora, tatpurusha,* and *ishana.* The inner significance of these names and their role and place in our spiritual unfoldment will be discussed in the commentary on the final sutra, sutra 4:34.

The anatomy of the mind and the samskaras pertaining to the yogis with afflictions in the dormant state are radically different from the anatomy of our mind. It is important to remember that the afflictions are samskaras—they have been manufactured by our mind and are stored there. By the time the afflictions have been rendered inert, all other samskaras have also lost their potency.

As we will see in sutra 2:27, another term for this level of freedom is *chitta vimukti.* The literal translation of *chitta vimukti* is "freedom from mind," but this gives the mistaken impression that in this state we no longer have a mind. This state has also been described as *dagdha-bija,* literally, "roasted seed," but this gives the mistaken impression that all samskaras, including the fivefold affliction, have been incinerated. The truth is that neither the mind nor the samskaras created by it and stored in it can be destroyed. Instead, in this state of freedom, the mind and its samskaras are purified and transformed into pure shakti. The yogi has attained *sarva-bhava-adhishthatritva,* the capacity to be the locus of all samskaras. He has also attained *sarvajnatva,* the capacity to have full knowledge of all samskaras (YS 3:49).

Freedom from affliction is a great achievement. We lose neither our mind nor its contents; rather, this achievement is accompanied by an extraordinary transformation of the contents of our mind. The blinding effects of avidya, the disorienting effects of asmita, the binding effects of raga and dvesha, and the frightening effects of abhinivesha are transformed into pure shakti, the power to be and the power to become, and this shakti is fully aligned with chiti shakti, the boundless eternal intelligence of Ishvara. Due to this alignment, we are established in chiti shakti itself. After casting off our bodies, we are fully absorbed in chiti shakti. At the behest of divine will, we incarnate as free souls, with access to limitless samskaras and the ability to retrieve those we need to fulfill the work of the divine. We are able to live in the world and yet remain above it. Birth and death and the experiences that fill our life have no effect on our essential self.

Most of us, however, are far from being free of afflictions. We share a world afflicted with pain and sorrow. As a remedy, Patanjali delineates the fundamental causes of our pain, beginning with a description of avidya in the next sutra.

SUTRA 2:5

अनित्याशुचिदुःखानात्मसु
नित्यशुचिसुखात्मख्यातिरविद्या ॥५॥

anityāśuciduḥkhānātmasu
nityaśucisukhātmakhyātiravidyā ॥ 5 ॥

anitya, short-lived; *aśuci*, impure; *duḥkha*, suffering; *anātmasu*, different from soul; *nitya*, eternal; *śuci*, pure; *sukha*, happiness; *ātmakhyāti*, the experience of atman; *avidyā*, ignorance, false understanding

Mistaking short-lived objects, impurity, suffering, and non-being for eternity, purity, happiness, and pure being is *avidya*.

The concept of *avidya* is the most confusing principle in Indian philosophy. Some describe it as lack of *vidya*—knowledge—and others as incomplete knowledge. Still others call avidya perverted understanding. Some insist avidya does not exist, but at the same time insist it is the ground for the phenomenal world, a world that is mere illusion. Some proclaim avidya is a unique category of reality, one that is free from four extremes: avidya is not real; it is not unreal; nor is it simultaneously real and unreal; nor is it devoid of reality and unreality. All of these philosophers employ hairsplitting logic to describe the nature of avidya, and when entangled in the web of their own logic, they try to escape by calling avidya *anirvachaniya,* indescribable. Thus indescribability has become the standard description of avidya. From a practical standpoint, this leads nowhere.

Yoga has no room for these confusing theories, arguments, and counterarguments. According to Patanjali, avidya exists. It is as real as anything belonging to the world of our cognitions and arises from the same place as all of our other notions and cognitions. Like everything in the objective world, avidya has a twofold purpose: *bhoga,* fulfillment, and *apavarga*, freedom.

From the perspective of those caught in the cycle of samsara, avidya is a debilitating mental condition. It is *ashakti,* the essence of powerlessness. It saps our genius, empties us, and fills the void with a false sense of I-am-ness, attachment, aversion, and fear. Those who have acquired wisdom know avidya is the creation of our own mind. While using the mind as its residence, avidya exerts its influence on every aspect of our being and the world around us. It hides our essential nature and projects something altogether different in its place. At the same time, the spark of inner intelligence not veiled by ignorance contradicts this projection, providing an impetus to lift the veil and rediscover our core being. This sets up a tug-of-war between vidya and avidya, between the forces of knowing and not knowing—and we have been caught up in this war from time immemorial. According to Patanjali, this struggle ends only when we understand the dynamics of avidya and transform it into vidya.

We can unlock the mystery of avidya by understanding the purpose of the objective world and the force that brings it forward. According to Kapila, the founding master of Sankhya Yoga and the Sri Vidya tradition, creation embodies the living grace of the divine (*Tattva Samasa* 27). As explained in sutra 2:19, *prakriti,* the homogeneous state of primordial nature, is indescribable. It is the resting ground of everything within the scope of the phenomenal world and everything beyond. All forces and attributes of the universe—including the fundamental potency of time, space, cause, effect, the karmic tendencies and destinies of individuals, and the entire cosmos—reside in prakriti as sheer power. The compassionate intention of Ishvara stirs unmanifest prakriti, activating the intrinsic forces of sattva, rajas, and tamas. This is followed by the manifestation of the world composed of matter and energy in an infinite array of shapes and sizes. As part of this manifestation we emerge from the timeless slumber of death. Our state of non-being is transformed into being, and we acquire our mind, senses, and all our karmic belongings, including avidya. We start a new life.

Our birth and the manifestation of the world have only one end: helping us fulfill life's purpose. In spite of this, religion and philosophy have described the objective world and our life in it as bondage. Across cultures and throughout history, religious and philosophical descriptions of the world are denigrating. The phenomenal world is said to be replete with misery and we come here as a result of our transgressions. The wisest course (so we are told) is to attain *moksha,* salvation, which in effect means extricating ourselves from the world as quickly as possible.

Patanjali's understanding and experiences are antithetical to this view. According to his predecessor, Kapila, the impetus behind our birth and the manifestation of the universe is *anugraha,* divine grace. Divine grace is suffused with unconditional love and compassion. *Purusha*, the intrinsic intelligence of prakriti, knows everything about each individual soul. Purusha knows the conditions of unfulfilled souls resting dormant in the absolutely subtle, vast field of prakriti. As purusha is spontaneously moved by its own realization, prakriti, the intrinsic shakti of purusha, begins to pulsate. This initial pulsation awakens numberless forces and resources, allowing the unknown to become known and the unseen to become seen. The world that was rendered imperceptible by the forces of dissolution now becomes perceptible.

Compassion is the sole cause of the initial pulsation—the power of compassion is itself the pulsation (*anugraha shakti*). Thus spiritually speaking, the power of compassion is our origin. Following *satkaryavada*—the cardinal doctrine of Sankhya Yoga, which holds that the cause always remains present in the effect—we see that every nook and cranny of our personal life, as well as the entire universe, is pervaded and sustained by the power of compassion. The sun shines due to the power of compassion inherent in it, and we thrive due to the power of compassion inherent in us. This power of compassion is the power of the divine. Avidya also has its source in compassion and is kept alive through its sheer power. In the final analysis, therefore, avidya is not a frightening adversary. Avidya is an affliction only because we do not know what it is. As soon as we know its source and its true nature, it is no longer avidya but pure shakti, the revealing power of pure consciousness.

Most philosophical texts have ignored the benevolent dimension of avidya. As explained briefly in sutra 2:1, when we awaken from the timeless slumber of death the first thing that comes into view is Ishvara, the lord of all beings, the intrinsic intelligence of prakriti. We see ourselves bathed in the life-giving light of Ishvara. We are brimming with joy at seeing our eternal companion, protector, and provider standing before us, inside us, and all around us. We are grateful to have found our self, our mind, and our senses.

The instant we become aware of our mind, however, we become aware of everything stored in it. The infinitely vast field of subtle impressions, habits, unfulfilled desires, likes, and dislikes is now in full view of our consciousness. With our rebirth, everything we acquired before is also reborn. Our prejudices, preoccupations, and preferences return. The mixed forces of doubt, fear, anger, hatred, desire, attachment, arrogance, lust, love, kindness, and compassion churn our mind. We are caught in the whirlpool of our mental contents. Our numberless and long-cherished mental tendencies begin to dominate our mind just as they did before. Our focus shifts from Ishvara to our inner turmoil. We become more interested in chasing our unfulfilled desires than in holding tightly to our eternal protector and provider. In short, we abandon Ishvara in favor of reclaiming our karmic belongings. Thus we are back in the same state of mind we were in when we took our last breath in the previous life. Yet divine grace does not abandon us.

The *Bhagavad Gita* tells us, "I [Ishvara] am well established in the heart of all beings. From me ensue memory and knowledge and the power that veils memory and knowledge. I am the one to be known. I am the creator of the means of knowledge and I am the knower" (BG 15:15). Knowing everything about ourselves while Ishvara remains in our full view is the greatest joy. But once we are separated from our protector and provider, knowing everything about ourselves becomes the source of our greatest misery. That is why the loving grace of the divine puts a veil over memories that serve no purpose in the life about to unfold. Divine grace does this by awakening our deep-seated avidya, the force that shrinks our comprehension and discernment.

Avidya enables us to draw a boundary around our self-identity. Due to avidya we have limited knowledge of our true self, our mind, our samskaras, and our destiny. As soon as we are born, avidya helps us identify with our body. Our spiritual and physical dimensions become intertwined, and our consciousness is confined to our biological and emotional needs. Our world shrinks to the size of our mind and its contents; we use our body to find safety and security within the confines of that contracted world. Our intelligence now flows through the narrow conduit of our body and sense organs. Even so, the bandwidth of our intelligence is enormous compared to many other species. That is why we are able to comprehend the difference between our body and pure consciousness. We are able to distinguish vidya from avidya, a subject Vyasa elaborates on in his commentary on sutra 4:33.

Figuratively speaking, we are half-enlightened beings. In part we are aware of the perfection and self-luminous nature of our core self, yet we firmly believe we are not complete without the objects of the world. Our intrinsic intelligence compels us to seek eternity, while avidya forces us to seek it in the world belonging to our body and mind. The pristine nature of our consciousness compels us to rediscover our intrinsic purity, but avidya forces us to seek it in the world stained by our likes and dislikes. The voice of our soul tells us the joy of our core being is unconditional and unbound, but avidya forces us to seek joy through the limited conduit of our senses. Similarly, our intuitive wisdom tells us that our body is not our soul, but avidya forces us to believe it is.

In commenting on this sutra, Vyasa says, "Avidya is neither valid nor invalid. It is simply contrary to vidya, correct understanding." As incorrect understanding, avidya is as real as vidya, although its function is totally opposite—avidya and vidya lead to two quite different experiences (*Isha Upanishad* 10–11). Avidya cancels the revealing quality of vidya; thus the experience it brings leads to bondage. Vidya cancels the veiling quality of avidya; thus the experience it brings leads to liberation. The light of vidya, intuitive wisdom, shines forth in proportion to the attenuation of avidya, the fundamental force of affliction. In other words, the veiling effects of avidya are attenuated in direct proportion to the radiant light of intuitive wisdom. We are neither fully under the influence of avidya nor are we fully enlightened.

As humans, we have the capacity to see the difference between avidya and vidya. We can choose to harness one and subdue the other and thus become the creator of our own destiny. Harnessing the revealing power of vidya and attenuating the veiling power of avidya is our unique human privilege. The failure to exercise this privilege breeds a long chain of afflictions. The first of these is asmita, the subject of the next sutra.

SUTRA 2:6

दृग्दर्शनशक्त्योरेकात्मतेवास्मिता ॥ ६ ॥

dṛgdarśanaśaktyorekātmatevāsmitā ॥ 6 ॥

dṛk, perceiver; *darśana,* perception; *śaktyoḥ,* power of; *ekātmateva,* apparent oneness; *asmitā,* false sense of self-identity

Asmita **arises from the apparent oneness of the power of the perceiver and the power of perception.**

A*smita* is the false sense of self-identity. It is the first step toward the concretization of avidya, false understanding. Asmita arises as avidya lays the foundation for a new reality parallel to the world created by primordial nature.

In Sankhya Yoga, the world that manifests from primordial nature is known as *bhautika sarga.* This world is made of our pristine mind and its various faculties, our senses, the five gross elements, and their corresponding subtle elements. It is endowed with nature's infinite richness. We are brought to this world to find our life's purpose: lasting fulfillment and ultimate freedom (YS 2:18). Every object and experience belonging to this world is infused with *darshana shakti,* the power of perception. The world created by primordial nature enables us to see ourselves as purusha, the perceiver. In other words, the world created by nature is meant to reveal itself to us, and this revelation allows us to see ourselves clearly.

Avidya disrupts this natural process by throwing a veil of confusion over our consciousness. We no longer see ourselves as a seer nor do we see the world as a conduit for revelation. This provides an opening for disbelief in ourselves—the strongest of all samskaras—to come to the forefront of our consciousness. Yet the memory of ourselves as pure consciousness forces us to doubt our disbelief in our true identity. This combination of confusion and doubt in our disbelief is the ground for the birth of a compromised self.

This compromised self is asmita, distorted self-identity. It is neither fully unreal nor fully real. It is neither completely free nor completely in bondage. It is neither completely enlightened nor completely ignorant. It is neither the same as pure purusha nor totally different. It is a confused state of consciousness, unsure of its true identity. Its intentions and actions are smeared with confusion. As asmita matures, its belief in its distorted understanding of itself also matures, until it altogether overshadows the experience of our true nature. This how a new reality—asmita—emerges from avidya.

The literal meaning of *asmita* is "the essence of I-am" or "I-amness." In the words of Patanjali, asmita is a mixture of the power of the perceiver and the power of perception. Asmita arises when consciousness, the perceiver, mistakenly identifies itself with the tool it uses to perceive objects. The mind is that tool. The mind is originally endowed with the power to perceive the world created by nature as well as the world created by itself. Asmita emerges when consciousness identifies itself with the mind and the objects experienced by the mind.

Consciousness is intrinsically pure and boundless. It is self-contained. Its intrinsic attributes—existence (*sat*), self-awareness (*chit*), and joy (*ananda*)—are not dependent on anything. This raises a question: Why does consciousness identify itself with the mind and the objects of the world and become dependent on them? Because of avidya—a mysterious force incomprehensible to an ordinary mind. We do not know when and how this mysterious force first cast its veil over our consciousness, so we refer to it as beginningless. Thus avidya's first descendant—asmita—is also beginningless.

Each time we are born, our asmita returns with all of its belongings—deep disbelief in the pure and pervasive nature of consciousness, deep belief in its own limited power and wisdom, and deep belief that its existence is dependent on worldly objects. This disbelief in the pervasiveness of consciousness, coupled with a strong belief in the existence of the objects of experiences, is avidya, the root cause of all afflictions.

Avidya has been nurturing our asmita from time immemorial. The samskara of this nurturance is stored in our asmita. Asmita has long been defending itself from all-pervasive, omniscient, omnipotent, and omnipresent consciousness. It has been fleeing from Ishvara, our primordial companion, guide, and protector. The samskara of this behavior is also stored in our asmita. These samskaras have made us comfortable with seeing ourselves as a distinct entity. We want to remain distinct. We have memories of being the lord of our little world and we yearn to remain the lord of that little world. The thought of losing our long-cherished lordly status and adopting a new identity is traumatic.

We are accustomed to living in a world defined by and confined to the forces of time, space, and the law of cause and effect. Our deep familiarity with ourselves as a limited entity makes embracing our limitless self extremely distressing. We prefer becoming "big" in our familiar little world to losing ourselves in the vastness of our pure consciousness. Thus we shun our *brahma bhava,* the all-pervading experience of consciousness, and instead embrace *jiva bhava,* the limited sense of individuality. *Jiva bhava* is another term for asmita.

To reiterate, asmita causes us to turn a blind eye to the purity and expansive nature of our consciousness. Instead of seeing ourselves as pure consciousness, we are aware only of our limited identity, which is composed of the subtle impressions of the past. These samskaras, under the leadership of avidya, bring forward our deep distrust in our own eternity, omniscience, omnipotence, and omnipresence. They force us to believe we are transient beings with limited knowledge and capacity. On the firm foundation of this belief, asmita creates an immensely vast and variegated world known as *pratyaya sarga*, the world of cognitions and re-cognitions.

We now see the world through the lens of our asmita. The samskaric properties of this false self-identity create a world filled with friends and enemies, virtue and vice. Asmita leads us to experiences of success and failure, gain and loss, honor and insult, and burdens us with inferiority and superiority complexes. Our inner luminosity becomes dim and (figuratively speaking) purusha, our inner intelligence, becomes blind. This blind fellow now seeks help from nature, which has been rendered lame by our avidya-driven belief system. The endless miseries that fill our life arise from this union of the blind and the lame. We will continue to suffer until this union—grounded in avidya—is broken.

This is a general description of the dynamic of asmita and its mother, avidya. As humans we have the privilege of disrupting this dynamic and extricating ourselves from the torrent of sorrow it brings. Compared with other species, our veil of avidya is relatively thin. Consequently, our individuated consciousness is neither completely blind nor completely lame. We have the power to discern, decide, and act, as well as the ability to distinguish the real from the unreal and the good from the bad. Because our retentive power enables us to hold a long chain of events and their consequences in our mind, we have the ability to perceive how a series of causes leads to a distinct effect. We also have the ability to disrupt, change, modify, or even completely nullify the chain of causes and engender a desirable effect. We can decide what our *dharma* is, the force that infuses our life with sustainability and leads us to our highest good. We have the freedom to purify our entire field of I-am-ness, which includes our mind, senses, and the vast range of our mental impressions. By making proper use of our inner luminosity, which is not affected by avidya, we can assess ourselves accurately. We have the capacity to decide what we must renounce and what we must acquire. We have the capacity to stretch our shrunken asmita and begin to live in an expanded world, the world created by primordial nature and illumined by nature's intrinsic intelligence.

When we fail to exercise this unique human privilege, our asmita shrinks and we become smaller every day. But when we exercise it, we can purify our asmita and become a *mahatma,* a soul with expanded consciousness. Simply put, mindful use of human birth elevates us to higher rungs of consciousness while mindless use of human birth degrades us. How this degradation comes about is the subject of the next sutra.

SUTRA 2:7

सुखानुशयी रागः ॥७॥

sukhānuśayī rāgaḥ ॥ 7 ॥

sukha, pleasure; *anuśayī*, that which rests in; *rāgaḥ*, attachment or coloring

Affliction that has pleasure as its resting ground is attachment.

At the core we are pure consciousness. We are self-luminous beings. As discussed in the previous sutra, under the influence of avidya we identify ourselves with the mind, the conduit consciousness uses to experience the objective world. As our identification with the mind matures, we no longer see a distinction between mind and consciousness—we no longer see who is the seer and who is the instrument of seeing. We become less interested in knowing our essential nature and altogether disinterested in becoming established in it. Our attention shifts instead to serving our mental world and the sensory objects associated with it. This leads to the formation of *asmita,* a sense of self-identity grounded in confusion and fed by avidya.

Asmita is a powerful force. It is composed of the power of pure consciousness and the power of the phenomenal world, including the mind teeming with seemingly numberless samskaras. Asmita is constantly fed by *avidya shakti,* the power of ignorance. Asmita is our powerful and stubborn distorted self-identity. Its refusal to examine itself and to consider the possibility of a higher and less-restricted identity is unbending. Asmita takes pride in denying that it has any problems and tirelessly defends itself from everyone and everything, including Ishvara. It is allergic to change. Yet there is hope, provided we exercise our human privilege—the capacity to change the dynamics of our asmita and expand the scope of our consciousness.

Failure to exercise our human privilege allows avidya and asmita to further nourish each other, and as they do, the influence of avidya over our consciousness increases and our asmita becomes more unyielding. Our love for our asmita grows exponentially and, consequently, the internal and external worlds created by it become ever more real—so real in fact that we no longer see any reality beyond them. The world of our mental impressions defines what is real and what is unreal. In the light of these impressions, the objects in the external world appear to be pleasant or unpleasant. In their light we regard some memories as delightful and others as painful. Due to our long-cherished relationship with those memories, we long to remain in their embrace. Craving pleasant memories and the objects associated with them is *raga,* attachment, third in the chain of five afflictions. Craving unpleasant memories and the objects associated with them is *dvesha,* the fourth affliction.

The afflicting role of raga in our life is more vivid and easier to understand than the roles of avidya and asmita. Pleasant memories and the objects associated with them are a major factor motivating our thoughts, speech, and actions. Our pleasant memories induce us to visit our past again and again. They motivate us to acquire pleasurable objects and claim them forever. We believe providence is on our side when we acquire enjoyable objects—we feel fuller, richer, and blessed. When we lack those objects, we feel providence is against us and experience ourselves as empty, poor, and cursed.

When pleasurable experiences recede after running their course, we try to recapture and re-experience them. The more often we repeat this cycle, the stronger the attachment. The intensity of the attachment determines what is important, valuable, and therefore desirable. The power of attachment forces us to return to the objects of our desire again and again. It consumes the discerning power of our consciousness so completely that we see no difference between ourselves and our desire. Nor do we see a difference between desire and the objects of desire.

Attachment blends us with our desire and the objects of our desire—we become one with the world of our desire. When our desire or the objects associated with it are destroyed, we feel as if we are being destroyed. Preventing this becomes our life's purpose. Consequently, we keep attending the world made of our pleasurable experiences.

Until we curb this afflicting tendency, the world made of our samskaras—our mental cognitions and re-cognitions—will continue becoming firmer and more compelling. The firmer and more compelling the reality of this world, the fewer reasons we have to discover life's true purpose—lasting fulfillment and ultimate freedom.

Unpleasant memories grip our mind as powerfully as the pleasant memories do. The next sutra tells us what happens when we fail to avoid embracing unpleasant memories.

SUTRA 2:8

दुःखानुशयी द्वेषः ॥८॥

duḥkhānuśayī dveṣaḥ ॥ 8 ॥

duḥkha, pain; *anuśayī*, that which rests in; *dveṣaḥ*, aversion

Affliction that has pain as its resting ground is aversion.

Pleasant and unpleasant memories go hand in hand—we constantly revisit them. We justify clinging to pleasant memories but fail to recognize our habit of clinging to unpleasant ones. After all, why hold on to unpleasant, undesirable experiences and the pain and sorrow they cause? Yet under the influence of a mysterious force we appear to treasure unpleasant memories even more than we treasure pleasant ones, although we may not realize it. This mysterious force is *dvesha,* the fourth affliction.

Dvesha is loosely translated as "aversion," which connotes a sense of dislike toward an object, an experience, or a feeling. It is a reaction to something—a person, an object, or an event—we hate. But in Sanskrit, *dvesha* carries more weight—it is a force accompanied by the desire to eliminate the object of our hatred.

Dvesha is a condition of mind that has no tolerance for an enemy. It is accompanied by the desire for vengeance and contains a strong element of violence. Dvesha captures and occupies our consciousness so powerfully that we cannot pull the mind away. Like raga, dvesha gives our asmita a sense of fullness. In the same way attachment prompts us to renew and rejuvenate pleasant memories, hatred prompts us to renew and rejuvenate unpleasant ones. This is why we have a hard time letting go of the things we dislike the most.

The truth is that what we do not want to let go of is dvesha itself. There is a strong tendency to protect and preserve the samskara of dvesha. In its presence we are compelled to find an object on which we can focus this afflicting force. If such an object is not available, we create one. Living without an enemy is as hard as living without a friend. Conquering an enemy in the external world is as glorious and empowering as forming an alliance with a group of loyal friends. Asmita loves glory and power, and dvesha is there to feed it.

Dvesha—hatred armed with anger, vengeance, and violence—is deeply debilitating. It drains the brilliance of our mind and sucks the vitality from our body. We go on harboring this debilitating condition as long as our body and mind cooperate. We attribute the pain caused by dvesha to external sources. We deny we are possessed by hatred and instead claim to hate only a particular person or circumstance. We insist there is a good reason for this. In short, we rationalize our hatred, anger, vengeance, and violence. But no matter how cleverly we veil it, dvesha destroys our inner peace. It dulls the brilliance of our mind, damages our faculty of discernment, and deranges our senses. Dvesha causes us to become irrational. It shakes our nervous system, disrupts the functions of our body, and eventually makes us ill—physically, mentally, and spiritually.

Dvesha, coupled with raga and fed by asmita and avidya, prepares the ground for the fear of death, the fifth and last affliction. That is the subject of the next sutra.

SUTRA 2:9

स्वरसवाही विदुषोऽपि तथारूढोऽभिनिवेशः ॥९॥

svarasavāhī viduṣo'pi tathārūḍho'bhiniveśaḥ ॥ 9 ॥

svarasavāhī, that which carries its own essence; *viduṣaḥ*, of a wise person; *api*, even; *tathārūḍhaḥ*, riding in that manner; *abhiniveśaḥ*, fear of death

Fear of death carries its own essence and rides [the consciousness] of even the wise.

Since the beginning of time, death has been shrouded in mystery to all but the yogis. Yogis see death and birth in the same light. With death, life passes from manifest to unmanifest; with birth, the unmanifest becomes manifest. Death has no power to destroy the essence of life—it remains the same in both birth and death. Death simply frees us from an old garment—our torn and tattered body and our relationship with the world dependent on our physical existence. Wise and capable yogis cast off their bodies as voluntarily as the rest of us change garments. To them, death is an opportunity to leave the past behind and prepare the ground to welcome newness. For most of us, however, death is devastating.

Fear of dying and clinging to life are two sides of the same coin. They carry equal weight. Memories pertaining to birth and death are reinforced each time we are born and each time we die. While we are alive, most of our actions are directed toward ensuring a long life—we wish to live forever. The samskaras of those actions and wishes are stored in our mind. Yet we die each time we are born. Death shatters our wish to live forever—we die against our will. The samskara of shattered hope is also stored in our mind. As we are taking our last breath, the life force presents our fading consciousness with a summary of our life, one that is virtually identical for most of us: life has been a pointless saga. And so we breathe our last with a feeling of deep regret. The samskara of this regret is deposited in our mind, and with this mind we are reborn.

At birth, the samskaras of our previous lives and deaths return. When we take our first breath we become aware at a subtle level of everything we experienced before. The most powerful of those experiences is the memory of dying while clinging to life. We know life is precious and we must protect it from death; we also know death is unavoidable. These two mutually supporting realizations fill us with fear, and so fear enters our life the instant we are born. It is accompanied by a sense of powerlessness because we know we cannot protect ourselves from death. Yet our strong desire to live compels us to deny this painful fact.

The knowledge that death is inevitable and our denial of it are deeply engrained. They are the grounds for our most primitive instinct—fear of death and clinging to life. This is the most vivid and active form of avidya. As we die, our asmita, raga, and dvesha are clumped into this vivid form of avidya. All feelings merge into the experience of dying—it is our final memory. This memory, which is the resting ground of our asmita, raga, and dvesha, is kept alive by the mysterious power of avidya, and so remains active even when we are disembodied. When life comes to an end, death comes to life. In the realm of death we are enveloped by fear. Birth gives us the opportunity to free ourselves from this numbing affliction.

The process of emerging from death and returning to life is at once simple and complex. According to Vyasa, the same force that led us to death brings us back to life. Avidya that has matured into asmita, raga, and dvesha is vivid in death, and avidya is the doorway to birth. In the realm of death, the entire range of avidya—including fear of death and clinging to life—is very much alive. As Vyasa explains in sutra 2:3, its subtle pulsation creates the atmosphere for our rebirth. It pulsates as *shakti matra,* sheer power, awakening and accelerating the functions of the three intrinsic attributes of nature: sattva, rajas, and tamas. This accelerated activity in the realm of the three gunas lays the foundation for change, and on this foundation the currents of cause and effect become connected. Once the forces of cause and effect are supporting each other, our karmas begin to bear fruit. As a result, we become aware of our existence and the life we experienced before. This awareness is infused with the memory of our past in which the final memory of fearing death and clinging to life figures prominently. Thus life begins again where it ended.

Fear of death and clinging to life are inextricably intertwined. They are at work when we are growing as a fetus—our brain develops in response to the demands of this primordial instinct. Fear of death and clinging to life establish themselves in the area that houses our limbic system, amygdala, and hippocampus—the region known as the primitive brain. Urges such as hunger, sleep, and procreation are an offshoot of the urge for self-preservation. While we are in the womb, fear is more in the forefront of consciousness than clinging to life. But soon after we are born, we begin to identify with our body, and clinging to life takes its place alongside fear in the forefront of our mind. The urge to live and the desire not to die exhibit themselves even when we are infants. Patanjali calls this urge a full-blown affliction, *abhinivesha.*

Abhinivesha is a composite of *abhi, ni,* and *vesha.* As a prefix, *abhi* means "from every direction, from every vantage point"; *ni* means "completely, without exception, in every respect"; *vesha* means "penetrating, piercing." Thus in the context of this sutra, *abhinivesha* means "the affliction that has penetrated every nook and cranny of our existence, influencing every aspect of our life." Its far-reaching effects can be seen from every direction and from every vantage point. No one is exempt.

Patanjali's use of *abhinivesha* is highly significant. In Sanskrit, the most common term for death is *mrityu* and the most common term for fear is *bhaya*. Here he avoids using *mrityu-bhaya* and uses *abhinivesha* instead. In doing so, Patanjali is telling us that fear is not an ordinary emotion nor is the memory pertaining to death an ordinary memory. Fear of death is an overwhelming experience. Before we die, we employ all our faculties to resist death but one by one our limbs and organs fail. The senses dissolve into the mind. Lacking support from *prana shakti*, the mind surrenders to death. Our consciousness fades and our existence dissolves into primordial prakriti. This destroys everything we once owned. It annihilates all the objects we employed to satisfy our cravings and plunders our highly prized asmita, the ground for our autonomy.

Death contains the memory of everything we have just lost, as well as the intense pain caused by this loss. When we are reborn, the memory of this intense pain awakens. In other words, the memory of death and the intense pain that accompanies it is established deep in our core. From here it spreads concentrically until it fills every aspect of our consciousness. It walks with us through every stage of life, but becomes fully manifest only after it has finished drinking the sap of our life.

As we grow, death grows along with us. We do not notice exactly when we become adolescent, adult, or elderly, nor do we notice the lengthening shadow of death. We do not see the connection between disease and aging or the connection between aging and death. If the realization dawns that we are aging and thus coming closer to the final moments of our life, we push it aside. According to the yogis, active dismissal of this realization is avidya.

We have formed a strong habit of embracing avidya tightly. The more tightly we embrace it, the duller, denser, and more inert we become. Our distorted sense of self-identity becomes ever more deeply entrenched. Our sense of I-am-ness becomes confined to our body and the world surrounding us. Our capacity to stretch the scope of our mental world and see the reality beyond our existing belief system declines. Our notions of safety, security, achievement, prosperity, dignity, power, and prestige become confined to our circumscribed world. Meeting the demands of the primitive urges of hunger, sleep, sex, and self-preservation becomes our priority. We are subdued by our subhuman tendencies—for the most part we are guided by our primitive brain.

The greater the influence of avidya, the duller and denser our inner faculties become. The flow of our inner intelligence is blocked. Communication among different organs of our body slows or even stops completely. This leads to a drastic decline in our power of discernment. We see things only in fragments. Our self-trust, the cornerstone of our life, crumbles. Loss of self-trust causes us to lose trust in our loved ones, providence, truth, and justice. Our enthusiasm for life evaporates. We become weak and pitiful. Our survival issues intensify until we are totally consumed by the urge for self-preservation.

According to the yogis of the Sri Vidya tradition, at this point *raudri shakti*, the forces governing the functions of the *manipura chakra*, become imbalanced. Pranic forces go haywire, disrupting the flow of the body's natural healing power. The connection between our abdominal brain and cranial brain (more precisely, the limbic system) is broken. The innate wisdom flowing through the vagus nerve is blocked, leaving our visceral organs undernourished and without guidance. Weak and dysfunctional organs are a breeding ground for disease. Because our innate wisdom has declined, diseases taking root in our internal organs and the deeper systems of our body are likely to go unnoticed. By the time they manifest, our vitality has been depleted and our body weakened. Our strength, stamina, and energy drain away and we begin growing old.

Old age is as mysterious as death itself—it walks into our life unannounced. Yogis regard disease and old age as death's lieutenants. To understand the dynamics of death it is helpful to take a closer look at the power of these lieutenants.

When Patanjali lists the nine obstacles to well-being and spiritual unfoldment in sutra 1:30, disease is first and foremost. He tells us that once we are in the grip of disease, the other eight obstacles—mental inertia, doubt, carelessness, sloth, inability to withdraw from sense cravings, inability to reach the goal (samadhi), and inability to retain it—come into play. According to the Sri Vidya masters, these obstacles lead to eight conditions: *alasya,* torpor; *kripana,* inability to let go; *dina,* self-pity; *vinidra,* disturbed sleep; *pramilika,* restlessness; *kliva,* powerlessness; and *nirahankara,* lack of self-trust. These eight conditions turn our body and mind into *vighna-yantra,* a machine that generates obstacles ("Lalitopakhyana" of the *Brahmanda Purana,* 7:38). They force us to work against ourselves, and the crippling conditions wrought by them accelerate the aging process.

The Sanskrit word for old age is *jara,* literally "that which makes us disintegrate; that which breaks us down." Old age is a process of deterioration. It demolishes our ability to deny we are running out of time. It took us a long time to build our self-image; we now see it vanishing and are powerless to stop it.

That is painful. Our youthful beauty and vigor were once a source of pride—they filled us with enthusiasm and confidence. As old age progresses, all this crumbles. Old age shatters our belief in ourselves. We begin doubting our long-held convictions and start questioning whether anything we have done in the past and anything we are doing now has any meaning. A feeling of purposelessness clouds our consciousness.

Old age enters the mind in the form of worry. As the yogic expression goes, "A funeral pyre consumes only the dead, but worry consumes the living." The effect of worry is far-reaching and devastating. Worry causes our neurons to fire incessantly and crushes our heart with its weight. Our power of concentration deteriorates. The ejection fraction of our heart declines. Our lung capacity diminishes and our breath is labored. We become restless, tense, irritable, and lonely. Worry forces our mental energy to flow outward. We become forcefully connected with the things we are worried about and disconnected from ourselves. At a subtle level, this disconnect tosses us into a void.

This void is the breeding ground for a variety of mental conditions that accelerate aging and render us increasingly weak and helpless. It quickly fills up with fear and doubt. Our insecurity intensifies. We become overly protective. The tendency to conceal and hoard our possessions strengthens. We are tired of living with emptiness but we have neither the strength to pull ourselves out of it nor the courage to share it with anyone. We are caught between wanting and not wanting. We want to be part of the world; we do not want to be part of the world. We want to live; we do not want to live. The world outside us is constantly evolving and demanding we change along with it, but the world inside us resists change.

An aging mind equates change with the loss of freedom. That is painful. Furthermore, the aging mind crying for freedom is continuously assaulted by asmita, raga, and dvesha. The power of asmita forces us to keep a tight grip on our self-identity. It impels us to fight and eliminate those who threaten our so-called freedom. The power of raga forces us to safeguard our possessions, both physical and mental, and not share them with anyone. The power of dvesha drives us to eliminate those who contest our ownership of our possessions. The closer we are to death, the more acute is our awareness of those we love or hate and of those who love or hate us. Our desire to reward or punish them also intensifies, but the circumstances accompanying old age leave us with little freedom to act. That is painful.

If we have not made a concerted effort to check our negative mental tendencies and have not transformed our mind, we become more judgmental, self-righteous, suspicious, and cynical in old age. A mind lacking radiance fails to process the flood of thoughts and emotions triggered by fear, anger, grief, and the feeling of powerlessness, and thus becomes increasingly confused.

We have been witnessing this pervasive condition of the final stage of life for thousands of years and have not yet been able to find a way out. That frightens us. Old age, with its frustrations, confusions, and uncertainties, ultimately delivers us to death. We were born, we grow old, and we will die—we know this. We also know we have not learned the art of staying young and transcending death. The knowledge of this undeniable truth—death—shakes us at our very core. Thus yogis call it an affliction.

When do fear of death and the other four afflictions come to an end? That is the subject of the next two sutras.

SUTRA 2:10

ते प्रतिप्रसवहेयाः सूक्ष्माः ॥१०॥

te pratiprasavaheyāḥ sūkṣmāḥ ॥ 10 ॥

te, they; *pratiprasava-heyāḥ*, that which is discarded or abandoned at death; *sūkṣmāḥ*, subtle

The afflictions are discarded at death only if they have become subtle.

Death and the fear of death come to an end when we succeed in attenuating and eventually destroying the samskaric seeds that motivate us to jump into the torrent of samsara, the cycle of birth and death. As we have seen, under the influence of avidya, asmita, raga, and dvesha, we cling to our mental possessions—our samskaras—reclaiming them life after life. Due to these afflictions, nothing seems more important than preserving our sense of I-am-ness, achieving what we like the most, and getting rid of what we hate the most. This brings us to this mortal plane again and again. In sutra 2:4, Patanjali tells us the strength and intensity of these afflicting tendencies determine how indiscriminately and impatiently we throw ourselves into the cycle of death and rebirth. The goal of yoga sadhana is to minimize the strength and intensity of these afflictions, so we can acquire the discrimination and patience necessary to break this cycle.

Some of us are totally obsessed with our mental possessions. We are convinced that the world around us is the only reality. The pairs of opposites—failure and success, loss and gain, insult and honor—are extremely meaningful to us. Sensory pleasures are our only source of fulfillment. Validation from outside sources is the foundation of our self-image and self-confidence. According to Patanjali, such people are bound to be consumed by fear. As he tells us in sutra 2:4, this is *udara,* the fully active form of affliction.

Some of us are less obsessed with our mental possessions. We understand life has a higher purpose, but this understanding is frequently interrupted by our long-cherished samskaras. We want to live in the light of a higher purpose, but our samskaras force us back into our old habits. We embrace a healthy lifestyle for a little while and then again fall prey to our habitual tendencies. This is *vicchinna*, the disjointed form of affliction. The majority of aspirants seeking lasting fulfillment and ultimate freedom are caught in this level of affliction.

Some of us are blessed with a higher degree of freedom from our mental possessions. We have reached a stage in our evolution where we are fully aware of life's purpose. This awareness is rarely interrupted by our samskaras; memories pertaining to the objects of our likes and dislikes remain, but they have no power to divert us from our quest. Causes of disturbance still exist, but we are not disturbed. As we walk through life, we are met with success and failure, gain and loss, honor and insult, but are unaffected by these experiences. Our afflictions have become *tanu*, attenuated, a level of mastery that comes from embracing a methodical mental discipline imbued with the principles of tapas, svadhyaya, and Ishvara pranidhana.

Even in their attenuated form, afflictions engender fear of death because some degree of clinging to life remains. The mind is not yet clear and still enough to sustain the experience of oneness with the primordial life force. Because a subtle craving to retain our self-identity remains, we resist becoming one with the primordial pool of life and its boundless intrinsic intelligence. But as we continue our sadhana, the subtle traces of this craving also evaporate. Our afflictions are purified and transformed—they become *prasupta*, dormant, and their binding qualities disappear. We reclaim our *buddhi sattva,* the essence of our mind. Our mental purity now equals the purity of pure consciousness. We have become *jivan-mukta,* liberated here and now.

This sutra—"the afflictions are discarded at death only if they have become subtle"—applies to those who have transcended the binding effects of avidya, asmita, raga, and dvesha. It applies to those whose mind is no longer stained by samskaras and who are thus established in their buddhi sattva. Their afflictions are purified and rendered dormant—so subtle they cannot be treated as "content." They no longer occupy mental space; they are absorbed in the mind and have become one with the essence of the mind.

In the yoga tradition this achievement is described by the terms *videha* and *prakritilaya,* and in the Buddhist tradition by the term *bodhisattva.* As long as these high-caliber souls are alive, however, they must abide by the laws governing their physical existence. At the physical level, they are still subject to hunger, thirst, and other biological imperatives. Their bodies retain their genetic characteristics even after enlightenment. Due to the intertwined nature of the body and mind, the innate memory of death and the fear pertaining to death remain. This memory finally comes to an end at the time of death. In their case, death brings complete freedom—they become *kavali,* absolutely free beings. The state of consciousness of such beings is called *kaivalya,* another term for *chiti shakti*, the intrinsic *prakriti* of pure consciousness (YS 2:27, 4:34).

At death, the purified, content-free mind dissolves into chiti shakti. This is a state beyond time, space, and the laws of cause and effect. In the truest sense, this is *asamprajnata samadhi.* It is the locus for liberated souls—this is where the yogis of this caliber live after they die. Their return to this world is an act of divine grace and the actions they perform are an expression of that grace. Their birth contains no trace of affliction. Their memory of their entire existence—past, present, and future—is at their disposal in a non-linear manner, yet they are untouched by their memories. Neither their birth nor their death nor the actions they perform between birth and death bear any karmic consequence (YS 4:30, 4:32–34).

Those of us who have not reached this level of spiritual accomplishment must work to attenuate the samskaras of our afflictions. How to accomplish this is the subject of the next sutra.

SUTRA 2:11

ध्यानहेयास्तद्वृत्तयः ॥ ११ ॥

dhyānaheyāstadvṛttayaḥ ॥ 11 ॥

dhyāna, meditation; *heyāḥ*, to be destroyed; *tat*, that; *vṛttayaḥ*, mental tendencies

The mental tendencies associated with the afflictions can be destroyed by meditation.

Samskaras—the drivers of our mental tendencies—manifest in the form of memory. We are able to remember something because the subtle impressions related to that object have been stored in our mind. Because they are hidden beneath thick layers of the forces of time, the mind is not aware of their existence. But like a seed that lies dormant until spring brings moisture and warmth, samskaras awaken when the conditions inside and outside the mind are conducive. Awakened impressions agitate the mind, demanding that it reach into the external world and find the objects with the potential to fulfill their needs.

In our day-to-day life we are quite aware of the objects of our thoughts, but mostly unaware of the thought process itself. Even when we pay close attention, it is difficult to trace the subtle sources of our thoughts. A careful analysis reveals that every thought construct or mental tendency is simultaneously connected both to the world outside and to the world inside. Objects in the external world have no power to agitate our mind unless this agitation is supported by deeper causes. Similarly, these deeper causes have no power to agitate our mind if the external atmosphere is not conducive. Some of our mental tendencies are fed primarily by conditions in the external world, while others are fed by deeply buried samskaras. Consequently, the mind's roaming tendencies seem to be originating from two different sources—external and internal.

When mental commotion arises from external sources, we can clearly see the relationship between cause and effect—both are gross and short-lived. Vyasa calls these mental tendencies *sthula,* gross—tendencies easy to comprehend and easy to manage. But when mental commotion arises from internal sources, we do not see the relationship between cause and effect—both are subtle. Vyasa calls such mental tendencies *sukshma,* subtle—tendencies difficult to comprehend and hard to manage. According to Patanjali, the mental tendencies belonging to both gross and subtle categories can be purified and brought under control through meditation.

Meditation is a powerful tool for mastering our mind and subduing its roaming tendencies. But meditation is itself a subtle process. As Vyasa states in sutra 1:1, a disturbed, stupefied, and distracted mind is not fit for meditation. For meditation we need a one-pointed mind, and if possible, one that is perfectly still. When the mind has become weak and responsive to sensory objects, it has no capacity to withstand the powerful storm arising from the realm of samskaras. Such a mind needs help. This is where kriya yoga comes in. With the assistance of tapas, we free our body of toxins and make it healthy, strong, and energetic, so it can support the meditative work of our mind. With the help of svadhyaya, we cultivate a positive and penetrating mind, so that we can clearly see the sources of our distractions, stupefaction, and disturbances. With the help of Ishvara pranidhana, we remain connected to our inner divinity and thus continue receiving nourishment for our soul.

Through kriya yoga, we eliminate our gross mental tendencies and free ourselves from the forces of the external world that drain our vitality and intelligence. The freer we are from the grosser forms of mental agitation, the easier it is to tackle the subtle forms. Ultimately, it is the subtle causes that throw our mind into a chaotic state. And the most subtle of these is the fivefold affliction: avidya, asmita, raga, dvesha, and abhinivesha. What happens when these powerful afflictions persist is the subject of the next sutra.

SUTRA 2:12

क्लेशमूलः कर्माशयो दृष्टादृष्टजन्मवेदनीयः ॥१२॥

kleśamūlaḥ karmāśayo dṛṣṭādṛṣṭajanmavedanīyaḥ ॥ 12 ॥

kleśamūlaḥ, that which has its roots in the afflictions; *karmāśaya*, reservoir of karma; *dṛṣṭa*, seen; *adṛṣṭa*, unseen; *janma*, birth; *vedanīyaḥ*, to be experienced

The reservoir of karma is rooted in afflictions and is to be experienced in seen and unseen lives.

Because karmas are stored in the mind, the mind is known as *karmashaya,* the repository of karmas. This is one of the cardinal concepts in the yoga tradition. *Ashaya* means "repository, sack, resting ground." The literal meaning of *karmashaya* is "karmic repository, karmic sack, the resting ground where our karmas are stored."

The ayurvedic system of medicine has several analogous terms. *Amashaya*, the stomach, is where our food (*ama*) is stored for digestion. *Malashaya*, the colon, is where waste matter (*mala*) is stored. *Mutra,* urine, is stored in the *mutrashaya*, the bladder. The only difference is that the karmashaya is integral to the mind, while the other "ashayas"—the stomach, the colon, and the bladder—are integral to the body. The condition of our body affects these organs, and the condition of these organs affects our body. Similarly, our general mental condition affects our karmashaya, and the conditions specific to our karmashaya affect the overall function and behavior of our mind.

Every organ in the body is endowed with unique powers and privileges, all of which are extremely subtle. We cannot observe them directly, but we can infer them by observing how the organ functions. Our karmashaya is subtle and its inherent powers and privileges are even subtler. However, we can infer the power of our karmashaya by observing its unique function. For example, we have all experienced how emotions arising from long-cherished habits override our rational mind, and so understand that our thoughts, speech, and actions have a powerful influence on our internal states.

Our experiences in this lifetime and in lives to come are outward expressions of what is occurring in the vast realm of our karmashaya. Our karmashaya is the lens through which we see ourselves and the world around us. Our major life decisions are made by it. Under its influence, we rationalize and justify our decisions. By and large, we do what our karmashaya tells us to do.

No action is perfectly pure or impure, perfectly good or bad; consequently, no karmic impression is perfectly pure or impure, good or bad. The impressions in our karmashaya—the building blocks of our personality—are of a mixed nature. As subtle impressions of our past virtuous deeds manifest, we are drawn toward virtuous actions, and when non-virtuous karmas manifest, we are drawn toward non-virtuous actions.

Karmic impressions influence our mental world. Impure actions reinforce impure karmic impressions, while pure actions reinforce those that are pure. Impure karmic impressions cloud our mind with desire, greed, confusion, and anger, and become the drivers of negative, destructive actions. Pure karmic impressions create a positive mental atmosphere, awakening virtues such as love, compassion, kindness, and selflessness, which then become drivers of positive, constructive actions.

This cycle gathers momentum as we go through life. If we are vigilant and have made a conscious decision to make a positive change in our lives, we consciously support our positive karmic impressions, while standing firm against the forces of those that are negative. But if we fail to use our power of discrimination—at whatever level it currently exists—and instead simply allow our karmashaya to dictate our thoughts, speech, and actions, we waste the precious gift of human life, and our past will continue reincarnating.

The law that good deeds bear good fruit and bad deeds bear bad fruit is both simple and complex. The causal potency of a karma is never destroyed. We do not always see the connection between our current misery and our negative actions nor the connection between our good fortune and our positive actions. When we do not see the connection between the cause and the effect, we attribute our current circumstances to destiny, God, or chance. But, according to both Patanjali and Vyasa, every action has a result and that result may be seen instantly, or it may be seen hours, months, years, or decades later, or even in a different lifetime.

All karmas fall into two major categories—*drishta-janma-vedaniya* and *adrishta-janma-vedaniya. Drishta-janma-vedaniya* means "the karmic result experienced in our visible life" while *adrishta-janma-vedaniya* means "the karmic result experienced in our invisible life." In other words, some karmas mature in our lifetime and others mature in lives to come. When actions bear fruit during our life span, we are often able to remember the nature of our actions and the conditions that led us to perform them. When we can see a direct relationship between cause and effect, we do not attribute the fruits of our actions to destiny, chance, or God. But actions we performed in a previous lifetime are outside the range of our memory. When such actions are maturing, we do not see the relationship between cause and effect and so attribute the cause to destiny, God, or chance. However, yoga philosophy assures us that the law of cause and effect regulates everything in both our inner and outer worlds—there are no accidents and no such thing as chance.

In commenting on this sutra, Vyasa explains why certain actions bear fruit in the same lifetime while others manifest in future lives. He tells us that the intensity of an action determines how quickly it will bear fruit. Devotion to Ishvara, divine forces, and the great seers is among the most potent of virtuous deeds. When accompanied by the intense practice of mantra, tapas, and samadhi, such action bears fruit in this lifetime. Spiritual practices of this nature—performed perfectly, sincerely, and intensely—create a highly distinct, spiritually charged karmic reality so powerful that it nullifies contrary karmas. Furthermore, the vibrancy of this newly created karmic reality stirs the vast field of our mind and the forces of nature in the external world.

As Vyasa explains in sutra 2:3, the stir created by this karmic reality sparks a fourfold action: the intrinsic forces of nature—sattva, rajas, and tamas—become animated; the condition for change is created; the currents of cause and effect are pulled together; and the secondary karmic strands of the past are awakened and employed to support the maturation of this newly engendered, spiritually charged karmic reality. This new reality ripens almost instantly and walks into our life, pushing aside the consequences of all other karmas. Vyasa gives the example of a dying young man, Nandishvara, who undertook an intense spiritual practice and not only defeated death but also rose to the rank of the celestial beings in that same lifetime.

Vyasa also gives an example of intensely bad karma and its quick result. Causing intense pain to someone who is fearful, diseased, or stingy engenders a highly distinct, negatively charged karmic reality. Betraying someone who trusts you or harming a high-caliber soul committed to intense austerity also engenders a highly potent negative karmic reality. This potent negative karma ripens quickly. Vyasa cites the example of a celestial being, Nahusha, who harmed Agastya, a high-caliber soul, and as a result, lost his place in heaven and became a reptile.

Vyasa reminds us that although we do not know what karmas we performed in our previous lives or when and how they are going to come to fruition in our current life, we still have a great degree of freedom to choose whether to live an ordinary life or an extraordinary one. We can surrender to the forces of "destiny" and accept what the cosmos presents or we can exercise our unique human privilege and aspire to an extraordinary life. If we commit ourselves to an intense and spiritually vibrant practice, as described earlier, we can create a potent karmic field that will nullify the effects of our negative karmas. We can break the fetters of our undesirable karmas and attain freedom here and now. What happens when we fail to do that is the subject of the next sutra.

SUTRA 2:13

सति मूले तद्विपाको जात्यायुर्भोगाः ॥१३॥

sati mūle tadvipāko jātyāyurbhogāḥ ॥ 13 ॥

sati, in the presence of; *mūle*, root; *tat*, that; *vipākaḥ*, fruition; *jāti*, species; *āyur*, life span; *bhogāḥ*, experience

As long as the root cause [the five afflictions] persists, karmas must bear fruit, and that fruition determines our birth in a particular species, life span, and life experience.

As stated in sutra 2:4, the afflictions exist in four states: dormant, attenuated, disjointed, and active. In general, our lives are the product of our active afflictions. The goal of yoga sadhana is to break the afflictions into pieces, attenuate their strength, weaken their effect, and eventually purify and transform them into *shakti matra*, sheer power. In this refined and transformed state, they carry neither positive nor negative traits. The memory pertaining to them is pure *buddhi vritti* or *jnana vritti* (Vyasa on YS 2:20). As buddhi vritti, they are the functional capacity of our buddhi, and as jnana vritti, they are the functional capacity of our knowledge. Thus in their most refined state, these so-called "afflictions"—avidya, asmita, raga, dvesha, and abhinivesha—are integral to our intrinsic luminosity. They are no longer afflictions. They are so fully purified that they are transformed into shakti matra, sheer power, and thus are part of our *buddhi sattva,* the essence of our intelligence. However, if the afflictions have not been attenuated and purified, then our karmas, which are rooted in the afflictions, will germinate, grow, blossom, and bear fruit. Our birth in a particular species, our life span, and the general experiences of pleasure and pain that walk into our life are the result of karmas rooted in fully active afflictions.

Questions invariably arise in regard to karma and rebirth: Is one karma the cause of a single birth or can one karma cause more than one birth? Are several karmas the cause of one birth or several births? After presenting a series of arguments and counter arguments in answer to these questions, Vyasa concludes that karmas are endless. They are of pure, impure, and mixed nature. Each karma has its own unique power and intensity. In regard to rebirth, one particular karma or group of karmas takes the lead and other karmas become subordinate. Vyasa reminds us that between birth and death we perform actions of all kinds—some good, others bad. Some are illuminating and others dulling. Some are uplifting and others degrading. Some make us feel proud and others ashamed.

The unalloyed brilliance of our inner conscience recognizes the overall quality of our lifelong actions. This recognition becomes vivid when we are dying. During our last moments, our limbs and organs fail, cortical activity declines, and linear cognition and thought processes collapse. At that time, the summary of our lifelong karmas and the experiences generated by them comes to the forefront of that aspect of the mind not dependent on our brain and nervous system. This is the totality of our mind, which, according to yogis, uses the heart and limbic system as its seat. What comes to the forefront of our mind when we are dying determines our next birth, *jati.* It also determines *ayu,* the length of our upcoming life, and *bhoga,* the general experiences of pleasure and pain accompanying that life.

Our current life is a continuation of our previous life, and that life was a continuation of the lives that preceded it. This seemingly beginningless journey is sustained by avidya, our active denial of our primordial relationship with the higher reality, coupled with our active desire to retain our false sense of self-identity.

What comes to the forefront of our mind when we are dying is not necessarily limited to what we have done and experienced in our current life but is the collective experiences of many lives, including the current one. If we are vigilant, we can comprehend this truth long before we die. Our primordial mother has invested us with her unsurpassed intelligence. It accompanies us day and night in the form of logic, reason, linear thinking, and the power of discernment. By employing this intelligence, we can design and implement a plan for attenuating our karmic impressions and reclaim our self-luminous mind. When we are breathing our last, our self-luminous mind will present our consciousness with an accurate and deeply fulfilling summary of life—life has been a beautiful gift. We will close our eyes with boundless gratitude, and this gratitude will become the locus for our consciousness after death. From here we re-emerge with the wealth of Ishvara pranidhana, trustful surrender, and *viveka shakti,* unshakeable power of discernment.

A key question remains: If our current actions and decisions are heavily influenced by our deeply rooted afflictions and the karmic impressions propelled by them, how much room is there to subdue or modify our karmic reservoir? Vyasa answers this important question by explaining there are two types of karmashaya: *niyata vipaka* and *aniyata vipaka. Niyata vipaka* means "karma whose fruition is fixed." As we saw in sutra 2:12, an action performed with intense force creates an intensely powerful karmic impression, which creates an irresistible karmashaya.

This distinctive karmic field is so powerful that it pulls supporting samskaras from the rest of the mind, while at the same time drawing support from the external world. Nothing can prevent the fruition of such karmas. An example of this kind of action is devotion to Ishvara, divine forces, and the great seers. This action is further intensified by the practice of mantra, tapas, and samadhi (YS 2:12). This kind of action and the resulting karmashaya supersede the fruition of all other karmas.

The second type of karmashaya is *aniyata vipaka,* "karma whose fruition is not yet fixed." This consists of a broad range of karmic impressions, some positive, others negative, and others of a mixed nature. None are powerful enough to override the effects of other karmas, although some are strong enough to take a leading role in their own fruition and in the fruition of weaker karmas of a similar character. Some of these samskaras are far from mature. Some are strong, while others are so weak they can be subdued by stronger ones or completely subsumed by an irresistible karmic impression.

In relation to this second type of karmashaya, we have enormous freedom to modify, alter, or nullify the karmic strands that result in rebirth, dictate how long we live in our body, and determine our general experience of pleasure and pain. What happens if we fail to exercise this freedom is the subject of the next sutra.

SUTRA 2:14

ते ह्लादपरितापफलाः पुण्यापुण्यहेतुत्वात्
॥१४॥

te hlādaparitāpaphalāḥ puṇyāpuṇyahetutvāt ॥ 14 ॥

te, they; *hlāda*, pleasure; *paritāpa*, sorrow or pain; *phalāḥ*, fruit; *puṇya*, virtue; *apuṇya*, vice; *hetutvāt*, due to the fact

They [karmas that result in rebirth, dictate how long we live in our body, and determine our general experience] are accompanied by pleasure and pain, for they are smeared with both virtue and vice.

As we have seen, no action is perfectly pure or impure, entirely positive or completely negative. Most of our actions are propelled by the false sense of self-identity, attachment, aversion, and fear. These four afflictions are rooted in avidya and nourished by it. For example, the virtuous deed of making a donation for cancer research is stained when it is made because a loved one died of cancer and we are afraid we too will die of it. The karmic impression of this action is mixed with generosity, grief, and fear. Although the good karma engendered by this charitable act will serve as a ground for happiness, it will be accompanied by pain because it is contaminated by the motivating factors of grief and fear.

The character of any karmic impression is largely dependent on the intentions behind our actions, which are almost always mixed. Our intentions are heavily influenced by our long-cherished likes and dislikes, which in turn determine what is pleasurable and what is painful. The desire to experience pleasure and avoid pain drives our actions. Desires are the extension of our self-identity, attachment, aversion, and fear of loss.

Samskaras stored in our karmashaya feed our desires. This stock of karmas does not distinguish good from bad or right from wrong. In its own mysterious way, this karmic stock triggers a taste for desirable objects. Pleasure comes from embracing the objects of our desire, and pain comes from being deprived of them. Because we all have our own unique tastes and interests, we have different desires. Our karmashaya is endless and so are our desires. Our pursuit of these endless desires has led us to fill this world with limitless objects.

We imagine that the more objects we accumulate, the better our chances of fulfilling our desires. Our body, mind, and senses are in the habit of fulfilling desires by consuming objects. There are two problems with this: first, the body and sense organs are finite and so is their capacity to consume; second, every desire and its corresponding object are invariably accompanied by a painful samskara. Thus every pleasure is accompanied by pain; every fulfillment is accompanied by a sense of emptiness. Yet lacking correct understanding and discernment, we continue chasing the objects of our desires. Desires destroy our peace of mind—and a mind devoid of peace cannot find happiness.

Peace comes neither from embracing objects of desire nor abstaining from them—peace comes from renouncing the desire itself. Renunciation of desire matures into happiness (BG 12:12). It cuts the karmic chain that begins with our karmashaya and ends by impelling us to perform new actions, which further strengthens the grip of our karmashaya on our mind. As the *Bhagavad Gita* tells us, renunciation of desires allows us to reclaim the essential brilliance of our mind. Our doubt about our true identity vanishes. Our retentive power, which contains our knowledge pertaining to our relationship with the highest reality, returns. As a result, we are neither attached to the objects of our desires nor averse to them; nor are we attached or averse to the actions associated with them (BG 18:10).

The influence of our karmashaya on our personality and overall thought process is so powerful that it seems impossible to swim against the current of our desires and nullify the force of our long-cherished samskaras. Even so, we must attenuate and eventually nullify the influence of our karmashaya to achieve lasting fulfillment and ultimate freedom. How to do this is the subject of the next sutra.

SUTRA 2:15

परिणामतापसंस्कारदुःखैर्गुणवृत्तिविरोधाच्च
दुःखमेव सर्वं विवेकिनः ॥१५॥

pariṇāmatāpasaṁskāraduḥkhairguṇavṛttivirodhācca
duḥkhameva sarvam vivekinaḥ ‖ 15 ‖

pariṇāma, change or effect; *tāpa,* distress or heat; *saṁskāra,* subtle karmic impression; *duḥkhaiḥ,* pain or sorrow; *guṇa,* intrinsic attribute of primordial nature; *vṛtti,* that which revolves; thought construct; *virodhāt,* because of contradiction or from opposition; *ca,* and; *duḥkham,* pain, sorrow, or suffering; *eva,* definitely or invariably; *sarvam,* everything; *vivekinaḥ,* a wise person

From the vantage point of a wise person, all is pain because everything is subject to change, distress, karmic impressions, and mutually contradicting forces of nature.

This sutra provides the key to comprehending the message of the *Yoga Sutra* and embracing yoga sadhana without deviation. Vyasa, who is known for his succinct and cryptic commentary, elaborates on this sutra at greater length than on any other sutra except 3:13 (which is an elaboration of *parinama,* the first word in this sutra).

Because Patanjali and Vyasa have spent so much time discussing the afflictions and the suffering originating from them, it may seem as if they are expounding the doctrine of suffering. They are not. In this sutra, both masters clarify the reasons for detailing the dynamics of suffering and explain how the knowledge of these dynamics can help us attain freedom from suffering once and for all.

Humans are amazing creatures. We have the capacity to train ourselves to perform incredible feats, one of which is to experience happiness when we are suffering. As a result, we manage to remain relatively oblivious to the pain and sorrow that fill our lives. We have adjusted ourselves to the experience of relative happiness—we are happy when painful conditions are relatively mild or when those around us are more miserable than we are. Seen through the lens of wisdom, this relative happiness is a delusion—it is actually sheer pain. Our shortsighted adjustment to relative happiness has impaired our desire to eliminate pain and its root cause. As a result, we search for quick fixes rather than a lasting solution.

In this sutra, Patanjali offers a contemplative tool for lifting the veil that blocks our awareness of the pervasiveness of pain. When this veil is lifted, we see we have been living in illusion—throughout life we have been defending pain itself, rather than defending ourselves from pain. This realization replaces our avidya, ignorance, with vidya, true understanding, impelling us to find permanent freedom from suffering and become established in our self-luminous and joyful essential nature.

The contemplative technique described in this sutra has four focal points: how everything is constantly changing (*parinama*); how our distress level (*tapa*) increases and habit (*samskara*) strengthens as we grow older; and how the forces of nature governing our internal ecology in a mutually supportive manner begin opposing each other as we move through life (*guna-vritti-virodha*).

Change (*parinama*) is the law of nature, yet we resist accepting its law. In early childhood we go with the flow. We are happy wherever we are—when we move to a new place it quickly becomes home. We are prepared to embrace change because deep within we are comfortable with the ever-changing ecosystem of our mind. The samskaras of our prejudices, preoccupations, likes and dislikes, and ideas of good and bad, vice and virtue, honor and insult, and success and failure have not yet manifested fully.

As we mature, our asmita, the sense of self-identity, also matures and our samskaras, coupled with avidya, feed our self-identity. As we begin to identify with our prejudices, preoccupations, likes, and dislikes, our understanding of vice and virtue gradually becomes inflexible. This inner rigidity prevents us from changing our ideas of honor and insult, success and failure. Internally we are frozen in time, while the external world continues to change. This leaves us with two options: renounce our ever-stiffening mental world and welcome change, or keep a tight grip on our rigid mental world and oppose change. Both are painful.

When changes occur against our will, it fuels the fire of anger (*tapa*). As we age, we become weaker, both physically and mentally. We no longer have the vitality, strength, stamina, and agility that were ours in youth. At some point, this reality hits us hard and it hurts. We feel entitled to enjoy the objects we earned through our hard work but our ever-weakening body and senses do not cooperate. That is painful. As we age, our patience declines. Our physical and emotional needs grow, while the relationships we counted on for support, love, and companionship disintegrate. That is painful.

Meanwhile, we continue performing actions, which are heavily influenced by habit (*samskara*), and so reinforce the samskaras that fueled them. In this way, *karma samskara chakra*—the cycle of action, to subtle impression, back to action—gains momentum. Through our current actions and habits, we are creating an environment conducive to the fruition of the karmas lying dormant in our karmashaya. With the exception of the karmas that are fully awakened and serving as a direct cause for our life span and the major course of our pleasant and unpleasant experiences, the fruition of karmas stored in our mind can be altered or even nullified to some extent. But most of us lack the vigilance that makes this possible. Our internal functions are programmed by our samskaras. We are like robots, engaged in thought, speech, and action in compliance with our programming. We invest our precious resources—our physical, mental, and spiritual energy—in reinforcing the power of samskaras, and thereby lose our opportunity to attain freedom here and now.

As long as the sap of life supports the normal functions of our body and mind, we comply with the inner calling of our samskaras. We engage in sensory activities and fulfill the cravings of our self-identity. We accumulate and consume. In our ignorance, we do not realize these charms and temptations are themselves consuming the sap of life. Eventually, our physical vitality and mental sharpness decline, but the call of our samskaras becomes louder because they have been continually reinforced. The senses demand more gratification, and our self-identity demands more recognition. But we are perpetually frustrated because neither our internal world nor the external world is supporting these demands. That is painful.

The fourth and last point of contemplation described in this sutra is the mutually opposing tendency of the gunas (*guna-vritti-virodha*). In sutra 2:3, Vyasa describes how karmic impressions buried in our mind are led to bear fruit. He tells us that the subtle pulsations of our karmas awaken and strengthen the intrinsic power of primordial nature. Nature's three forces become active, and their activity lays the foundation for change and connects the currents of cause and effect.

Our karmas mature only when the forces of nature begin to function in a mutually supportive manner. This occurs when we are awakening from the slumber of death. The force of sattva, illumination, enables us to become aware of ourself as a distinct being. Rajas, the force of activity, motivates us to experience ourself. Tamas, the power of inertia, puts a veil over our self-awareness. These three forces working together enable us to draw a boundary around our self-identity and inspire us to be born into the *jati,* species, most suitable to the fruition of our principal karmas. Furthermore, through their mutual cooperation, these forces determine *ayu,* the length of our life, and *bhoga,* the major course of our experiences.

A highly regulated mechanism ensures that the building blocks of our personality—sattva, rajas, and tamas—function in a well-balanced manner. When rajas is dominant, for example, we become active. If we do not slow down, we become depleted. To prevent this, tamas, the force contrary to rajas, becomes active. The dominance of tamas results in weariness, forcing us to slow down. But if tamas remains dominant for too long, we become inert and sluggish. In order to counter the negative effects of tamas, sattva awakens. This force of illumination and alertness pulls us out of inertia, thus again setting the stage for rajas.

An example will help us comprehend how these intrinsic forces of nature lead our karmas to fruition. When food reaches our stomach, enzymes rush to digest it. The heavier, more tamasic the food, the longer it remains in the stomach and the more bile—a fiery sattvic substance—is released by the liver. This cooperative interplay of sattva and tamas breaks down the molecules, making the nutrients available to our body. To use another example: In an emergency our sympathetic nervous system is triggered, accelerating the activities of the adrenal gland. This is a function of rajas. To control the adrenal rush, the sympathetic response is tempered by the parasympathetic nervous system. This is the function of tamas. The balancing act between rajas and tamas is due to sattva.

As we move through life, the mutual support of sattva, rajas, and tamas declines. For example, we are hungry but have no appetite. We are exhausted but cannot fall asleep. We are burdened by worrisome thoughts but cannot drop them. We are suffering from loneliness but cannot stand the company of others. Our intrinsic forces are no longer friendly with each other. The forces of light and darkness, stability and inertia are not cooperating. They are no longer comfortable with each other and that is making us uncomfortable with ourselves. That is painful.

As we have seen in sutra 2:9, the powerful urge for self-preservation—fear of death and clinging to life—forces us to believe that our familiar world is the only reality (*Katha Upanishad* 1:2:6). We are so preoccupied with the acquisition and preservation of short-lived objects that we have no time and energy for introspection: Where do we come from? Where do we go? What is the purpose of this endless cycle of coming and going? Living with pain and sorrow appears normal. Lack of knowledge regarding higher reality, and our long-cherished familiarity with our known world, have rendered us insensitive to the pervasiveness of sorrow and pain, so it never occurs to us to seek a permanent cure. We are comfortable with our relative happiness and have adjusted ourselves to the ongoing struggle. We accept mixed elements of love and hatred, cruelty and compassion, anger and tranquility as normal. Sickness is as integral to us as health. Our world is composed of this reality. We are born into this world, live in this world, and die in this world. Most of us do not see a reality beyond it.

According to Vyasa, yogis are highly sensitive to their own afflictions as well as to those of others. In fact, as Vyasa states, yogis are much more sensitive to afflictions than ordinary people. Due to their high degree of purity, they are acutely aware of the subtle causes of pain and sorrow. They have *samyag-drishti,* right vision.

They are able to see things correctly and completely. This correct and complete understanding is called *samyag-darshana.*

When they see an unwholesome karma stored in their karmashaya, yogis do not grieve or feel regret, nor do they feel a sense of pride upon seeing a good and auspicious karma. They acknowledge what they are and use their power of discernment to put their knowledge to good use. They make an effort to attenuate the potency of their unwholesome karmas and to further intensify the effects of their good karmas. Their pain arises from their inability to avert the forces of karmas that have already starting bearing fruit. They know these karmas determine their life span and the overall course of their pleasant and unpleasant experiences. They know they must ride their karmic roller coaster until these karmas run their course.

These yogis have another source of pain. Through their purified mind, they are able to see why there is suffering in the world. They know that much of it can be eliminated. But they also see how adamantly people are engaged in defending their pain instead of defending themselves from pain. They recognize that people have little or no trust in themselves and completely lack an understanding of higher reality. They see people continually reinforcing their unshakeable belief that the world of intermingled sorrow and joy is the only reality. These yogis know that the same principles that granted them freedom from the long chain of sorrow can help others escape the torrent of pain, but they also know that most people have no interest in those principles. Yogis find it painful to see their fellow beings suffering from their deeply rooted afflictions when a cure is readily available.

The more purified the body and mind, the more attenuated our afflictions. The more attenuated the afflictions, the thinner the veil of avidya. The thinner the veil of avidya, the more radiant the inner luminosity. The more luminous the mind, the greater the chance of having *samyag-darshana,* the complete vision and understanding of reality. Samyag-darshana demolishes the wall that stands between one's self-identity and the identity of others, and so the pain of others becomes the yogis' pain. The yogis have attained freedom from all forms of pain and its causes except those that ground them in their current physical body. They know they will be free even from those once they drop their body, and they wish for their fellow beings to experience the same freedom.

Long-forgotten actions, the subtle impressions of those actions stored in our mind, and the dynamic forces that govern and guide our destiny are almost impossible to comprehend. We know so little about the mysteries of our body, and even less about the deeper mysteries of our mind, karma, and rebirth. When generations of dedicated researchers cannot discover many of the secrets of our physical world, how can we discover a particular form of sorrow and its subtle cause and eliminate it once and for all? This is the subject of the next sutra.

SUTRA 2:16

हेयं दुःखमनागतम् ॥१६॥

heyaṁ duḥkhamanāgatam ॥ 16 ॥

heyaṁ, that which can be abandoned or renounced; *duḥkham*, pain, sorrow; *anāgatam*, that which has not yet come

Pain that has not yet come can be abandoned.

In sutras 2:12 and 2:13, Patanjali and Vyasa tell us our current life is the result of karmas performed in previous lives. In other words, our present is the product of our past—our current pleasant and unpleasant circumstances are the result of our previous actions. Some of these current circumstances are avoidable while others are not. Our *adrishta-janma-vedaniya karmashaya*, the reservoir of karmas to be experienced in unseen lives, guides us to take birth in a particular place at a particular time. These karmas are the building blocks of our destiny—the pain or pleasure resulting from them is unavoidable. When we are in our mother's womb, for example, we cannot avoid being affected by her habits.

But we do have a choice in regard to other experiences and circumstances. Patanjali calls these experiences *heyam*, avoidable. Actions that have not begun bearing fruit can—with effort and wisdom—be nullified. A simple example is avoiding the ill effects of poisonous food with a quickly administered antidote; the longer we wait, the less likely it is we will avoid being harmed. Or to give a more complex example: some of us are predominately vatic—nervous, unstable, and easily stressed—and therefore prone to hypertension, high blood pressure, and heart failure. These conditions can be avoided by adopting a vata-calming lifestyle: eating nourishing food, balancing the functions of the sympathetic and parasympathetic nervous system, and calming the autonomic nervous system with regular breathing exercises. These practices can be further strengthened with meditation and contemplative techniques, thereby avoiding many of the deleterious effects of a vata imbalance.

According to yoga, most of our sorrowful conditions are due to sheer carelessness. When an afflicting condition gains so much momentum that it becomes overtly painful, we look for a cure. At other times, we are so preoccupied by the demands of our self-identity, attachment, aversion, and fear that we fail to notice we have a problem. Pain warns us that the sap of life is draining away and we must do something to stop it. If we heed this warning, we can overcome the pain and eliminate the subtle conditions that are causing it. The subtle cause of suffering is the subject of the next sutra.

SUTRA 2:17

द्रष्टृदृश्ययोः संयोगो हेयहेतुः ॥१७॥

draṣṭṛdṛśyayoḥ saṁyogo heyahetuḥ ॥ 17 ॥

draṣṭṛ, seer; *dṛśyayoḥ*, of the seeable; *saṁyoga*, complete union; *heyahetuḥ*, the cause of pain

The union of the seer and the seeable is the cause of pain.

This is one of the most succinct and compact sutras. In conjunction with sutras 2:18–25, it constitutes the core of yoga metaphysics and philosophy. In a traditional setting, this sutra is taught only after clarifying the key concepts of Sankhya philosophy.

As ordinarily conceived, Sankhya philosophy posits two sets of absolute reality—purusha and prakriti. They are said to be entirely distinct: purusha is intelligent consciousness; prakriti is unintelligent matter, beyond any point of reference. According to this interpretation, there are numberless purushas but only one prakriti. Both sets of reality are beyond time, space, and the law of cause and effect. The phenomenal world ensues when these two distinct realities unite. Their union is intentional—purusha is in bondage and seeks prakriti's help in finding freedom. Although prakriti has all the tools and means for purusha's deliverance, she is unintelligent and does not know what she has and does not have. As a result, she cannot help purusha without purusha's help. When the two embrace, the phenomenal world comes forward. All the tools and means—including the objective world, made of an infinitely vast range of matter and energy contained in prakriti in unmanifest form—now become manifest. Purusha attains liberation using the tools and means that emerged from prakriti. Here liberation is defined as purusha isolating itself from prakriti, or vice versa.

In the traditional system of learning, we are led to identify five fundamental flaws in the foregoing interpretation of Sankhya philosophy. In the first place, there cannot be two absolutes, let alone a multiplicity of absolutes. Second, intelligent purusha is said to be in bondage and so needs help from unintelligent prakriti. This calls the intelligence of purusha into question. Third, the union of purusha and prakriti results in the manifestation of the phenomenal world, allowing the unmanifest tools and means of liberation to become manifest and thus accessible. By using these tools purusha and prakriti are pulled apart, and their mutual isolation results in freedom. But purusha and prakriti were already distinct and separate, and so were already free. What further freedom are they seeking by uniting only to separate again? Fourth, this interpretation of Sankhya philosophy is marred by a contradiction: the manifestation of the phenomenal world resulting from the union of purusha and prakriti is the source of bondage, but the same world is the source of liberation. Finally, when asked who exactly is in bondage, philosophers waver between purusha and prakriti.

The flawed interpretation of Sankhya described above is primarily based on a single text, the *Sankhya Karika*. We are able to formulate the more comprehensive philosophy Patanjali uses as the foundation for the *Yoga Sutra* only when we place the *Sankhya Karika* next to other prominent texts, such as the *Srimad Bhagavatam* and the *Bhagavad Gita*. This comprehensive philosophy is traditionally described as Sankhya Yoga. In the light of Sankhya Yoga, students trained in the Himalayan tradition are led to identify and resolve the five major flaws outlined above. Only then do sutras 2:17–25 become fully accessible.

According to Sankhya Yoga, the infinitely vast phenomenal universe is not the result of the union of numberless purushas with prakriti. Prakriti manifests as what we know as the phenomenal world through the unalloyed intention of one purusha (BG 9:10). That purusha is Ishvara (YS 1:24–26). Another name for Ishvara is *parama purusha,* the highest or absolute purusha. Prakriti is intrinsic to purusha; it is as intelligent and capable as purusha. Prakriti is purusha's own *svabhava,* its own inherent nature. Therefore, Ishvara and Ishvara's prakriti are one and the same. The phenomenal world, which manifests from prakriti, is as eternal and intelligent as prakriti itself. The *Bhagavad Gita* calls the manifest world Ishvara's own *vibhuti,* boundless excellence. This world is infused with *aishvarya,* the essence of Ishvara, and thus affords no room for sorrow. In this world individual souls are born, live, and die, only to be born again. These individual souls are called *purushas.*

Parama purusha or Ishvara is not an individual in any sense—it is unitary and universal. To distinguish this universal being from individual souls, Patanjali uses the term *purusha vishesha,* special purusha. Absolute freedom from kleshas, karmas, karmashayas, and the fruition of karmashayas, as well as absolute omniscience, are the intrinsic virtues of this special purusha (YS 1:24–26). It is the knower of itself. It is *akshara*, immutable. It is not subject to birth, death, decay, and destruction. These virtues are its svabhava. Due to its absolute pure nature, Ishvara's knowledge of everything that exists is utterly pure and pristine.

In contrast, we are individual purushas. Our individuality lies in the fact that we are smeared with kleshas, karmas, and karmashayas. Our knowledge is limited. We know ourselves only through a conduit—*buddhi*, the innermost faculty of our mind.

We are *kshara,* mutable. We are subject to change—birth, decay, and death. Numberless karmic impressions, including samskaras of the kleshas—avidya, asmita, raga, dvesha, and abhinivesha—constitute our svabhava. Due to the impurities inherent in our nature, our knowledge is limited, impure, and faulty.

We are not pure consciousness. We are a blend of consciousness and the conduit consciousness uses to experience itself—the mind. Because we do not know when consciousness and the mind became so perfectly blended, this union is described as "beginningless." In other words, *individual soul* refers to a unique form of reality in which consciousness and mind are indistinguishably intermingled.

Consciousness is not our creation and neither is our mind. What is our creation is the belief that our mind is consciousness. When this belief entered our consciousness is beyond our comprehension. It is described as avidya, ignorance, and is said to be beginningless. Avidya holds our consciousness and mind together (Vyasa on YS 2:24). Avidya is the mother of the entire range of afflictions—sorrow evolves from avidya and its offspring. According to Vyasa, "One who understands the trio of consciousness, mind, and avidya (the force that holds the two together) will adopt a preventive measure and thus will not suffer from sorrow." This preventive measure requires understanding the difference between consciousness (which is as pure, pristine, and omniscient as that of Ishvara) and the mind (which is smeared with numberless samskaras). This preventive measure also requires that we understand how the force of avidya distorts all our experiences, including the experiences of our inner being and the external world.

The mind is the repository of karmic impressions. In the *Sankhya Karika,* Ishvara Krishna calls them *bhavas* (SK 52). They give our mind a unique character. Samskaras are so perfectly absorbed in the mind that the two—samskaras and mind—have become one. As Vyasa tells us in sutras 4:19 and 4:23, the mind has no capacity to locate itself without samskaras. However, unless it locates itself, it cannot attain freedom from samskaras (SK 52). Because consciousness has identified itself with the mind and vice versa, we have no way of attaining freedom from the binding forces of our samskaras unless the samskaras manifest and become vivid. As described in sutra 2:3, when these samskaras awaken, they animate and intensify the functions of nature's intrinsic forces, set the stage for change, fuse the currents of cause and effect, and bring our karmas to fruition.

Karmic fruition is another term for the manifestation of samskaras. Karmic fruition stirs the entire mind field. Our thoughts, speech, and action are the outward expressions of karmic fruition. We can infer our subtle samskaras from their outward expression. By using the power of discernment, we can distinguish between uplifting samskaras and degrading ones. With patience and systematic practice, we can create more uplifting samskaras, and thereby nullify the effects of degrading samskaras. This enables us to reclaim the intrinsic luminosity of our mind. A luminous mind is infused with *viveka shakti*, the power to see itself as a conduit of the seeing power of consciousness, instead of seeing itself as the proprietor. This is freedom.

Freedom is possible only when our samskaras manifest vividly. This, in turn, is possible only when the seer and the seen (consciousness and mind) are united. As Vyasa says, the pain resulting from this union is *arthakrita*, purposeful. Attaining freedom from our long-standing pain is the purpose of the union of the seer and the seen. This union brings us to this world—a world that offers us everything we need to attain freedom from sorrow. That is the subject of the next sutra.

SUTRA 2:18

प्रकाशक्रियास्थितिशीलं भूतेन्द्रियात्मकं
भोगापवर्गार्थं दृश्यम् ॥१८॥

prakāśakriyāsthitiśīlaṁ bhūtendriyātmakaṁ
bhogāpavargārthaṁ dṛśyam ॥ 18 ॥

prakāśakriyāsthitiśīlaṁ, having the nature of illumination, activity, and stability; *bhūtendriyātmakaṁ*, composed of elements and senses; *bhogāpavargārthaṁ*, the purpose of fulfillment and freedom; *dṛśyam*, objective world

The objective world, composed of elements and senses and having the inherent properties of illumination, action, and stability, has a twofold purpose: fulfillment and freedom.

We are citizens of two worlds: the world created by primordial prakriti and the world created by us. According to *satkaryavada,* the cardinal doctrine of Sankhya Yoga (which holds that the cause remains present in the effect), the world created by primordial prakriti is imbued with all the qualities, characteristics, powers, and privileges intrinsic to primordial prakriti. Primordial prakriti is Ishvara's intrinsic shakti—it is divine and almighty. In the Sri Vidya tradition, primordial prakriti is known as *svatantrya shakti,* absolutely autonomous divine will.

Following that same cardinal doctrine, the world created by us is imbued with the inherent properties of our prakriti. Our prakriti is composed of our numberless samskaras and is as limited as we are. Each of us is characterized by our unique strengths and weaknesses and so is our prakriti. Because our consciousness is fragmented and our knowledge is conditioned by time, space, and the law of cause and effect, our prakriti is also fragmented and conditioned. Our prakriti has limited freedom of will—it is made of the binding qualities of our samskaras, and so the world emerging from it is characterized by bondage.

In this sutra, Patanjali describes the nature of the world evolving from primordial prakriti, while Vyasa explains how the resources available in the world of Ishvara can help us free ourselves from the afflictions inherent in the world we have created.

The phenomenal world is the creation of primordial prakriti, the intrinsic shakti of Ishvara. Everything—from waves of energy to subatomic particles, all the way to unimaginably vast galaxies and the senses that enable us to perceive them—has evolved from primordial prakriti. To convey the idea that this shakti is Ishvara's own power of creativity, philosophers use the term *prakriti*, literally "the supreme creative force." To convey that there is nothing beyond this power, philosophers use *pradhana*, literally "main"—the highest. Primordial prakriti is *aishvarya*, Ishvara's own essence. It is whatever Ishvara is, and Ishvara is whatever prakriti is.

The world perceptible to our senses and the mind through which we perceive it are the manifest form of unmanifest prakriti. It is imbued with all the divine properties of Ishvara. It contains everything prakriti contains—nothing less, nothing more. From a practical standpoint, Ishvara's intrinsic shakti consists of three mutually supportive powers: sattva, rajas, and tamas. In the tantric tradition, these powers are known as *jnana shakti*, unrestricted power of knowledge; *iccha shakti*, unrestricted power of will; and *kriya shakti*, unrestricted power of action. At a deeper, esoteric level, these powers are known as *aghora, ghora,* and *ghora-ghora-tara.* Like wetness in water and heat in fire, these powers are inherent in every aspect of the phenomenal world. Thus every object and experience is imbued with the powers of *prakasha,* revelation; *kriya,* activity; and *sthiti,* stability.

The human body is made of five gross elements: earth, water, fire, air, and space. These elements are not our creation but have evolved from primordial prakriti. We are made of the mind and the senses—all of which have evolved from prakriti. Our mind and senses are imbued with inner luminosity, which is not our creation but comes from primordial prakriti. Similarly, the world composed of matter and energy has evolved from primordial prakriti. Thus our body, mind, senses, and the phenomenal world are infused with the limitless creativity of primordial prakriti. To be born as a human and to live in the world of primordial prakriti is a blessing and a privilege, for it offers an opportunity to attenuate and eventually eliminate the world filled with afflictions, which are our own creation.

We have created our own little world parallel to the world of primordial prakriti. This self-created world is made of our samskaras, which are nourished by avidya, asmita, raga, dvesha, and abhinivesha. Sorrow is the underlying theme. The more confined our consciousness is to our self-created world, the more miserable we are. Birth in a human body gives us the opportunity to gather tools and means from the phenomenal world created by prakriti, which is untainted by our karmic impressions. By using these tools we can purify our self-created world and correct our distorted understanding of ourselves, the phenomenal world, its creator, and our relationship with the creator. This equips us to see that every object and experience belonging to the phenomenal world is meant for us. If used properly, everything in the world has the capacity to grant us *bhoga,* fulfillment, and *apavarga,* ultimate freedom.

Yogis in the Sri Vidya tradition explain why everything—from the minutest particle to the mightiest star—is capable of granting us fulfillment and freedom. Following the doctrine of satkaryavada, the infinitely vast range of powers intrinsic to Ishvara is passed on to everything in creation. Transformative power is the defining attribute of the phenomenal world—everything has the inherent capacity to transform itself and transform others. This manifests in countless ways. For example, *anima,* the capacity to be small, *mahima,* the capacity to be big, *garima,* the capacity to be heavy, *laghima,* the capacity to be light, and *vashitva,* the capacity to control, are inherent in every aspect of creation. The fundamental power of transformation confers the ability to be big, small, heavy, light, thick, thin, high, and low. It confers the ability to attract, repulse, react, unite, and disintegrate.

Because the transformative power of the divine pervades every aspect of the phenomenal world, it infuses our body, mind, and senses. Seeds sprout and unveil their inherent qualities and minerals unfold their medicinal properties because of this power. The science of medicine operates on the ground of the transformative power contained in both the medicine and the patient. The nuclear reaction at the core of the sun produces heat and light because the sun is endowed with the power of transformation. The laws of physics and the formulas of chemistry work because all matter and energy is infused with this power. Sacred rituals and spiritual practices arise from humankind's timeless experience that the space surrounding us is filled with the intelligent power of transformation. Transformative power is omniscient, eternal, and omnipresent.

While presenting the Sri Chakra model of yoga sadhana, the yogis of the Sri Vidya tradition made a comprehensive list of the shaktis continually engaged in bringing about transformation for the sake of our bhoga, fulfillment, and apavarga, freedom. The concept of bhoga and apavarga presupposes that every aspect of the universe is derived from the fundamental forces of sattva, rajas, and tamas, and is constantly propelled by them. As we have seen, these forces are the intrinsic properties of prakriti. They *are* prakriti—the divine shakti of Ishvara. Sattva, the force of illumination, rajas, the force of activity, and tamas, the force of stability, are at work simultaneously. In the scriptures, these shaktis are known as *aghora, ghora,* and *ghora-ghora-tara.* The yogis address them as "divine mother."

Numberless shaktis emerge through the mutually supportive interaction of sattva, rajas, and tamas, and are infused with their power. The yogis call these shaktis *matrikas,* mothers, for everything in the universe manifests from them. Thus all entities—sentient and insentient, small and large—are their children.

As her children we contain the revealing, pulsating, and grounding properties of our wprimordial mother, prakriti. However, in the long journey of life, we have accumulated a thick layer of karmic dust around our consciousness that impels us to perpetuate our self-created misery. As a result, we are unable to see and benefit fully from our inherent self-revealing, pulsating, and grounding attributes. Through tapas, svadhyaya, and Ishvara pranidhana we become more aligned with sattva and expand our inner luminosity. Eventually, we attain the revelation of our essential nature and become established in the divinity who pulsates as life.

The basic impetus behind the manifestation of primordial prakriti is the desire to awaken us—the individual souls—from the timeless slumber of death and put us on the path of fulfillment and freedom. This impetus is divine and pure. It is infused with unconditional love and compassion, which is why the world evolving from primordial prakriti arranges itself in a manner that leaves us no alternative but to attenuate and eventually demolish the self-created world of our afflictions. In his commentary on this sutra, Vyasa describes the process whereby prakriti empowers us to find our life's purpose—bhoga and apavarga, fulfillment and freedom. Because this topic is so crucial for our inner quest, both Patanjali and Vyasa return to it repeatedly (YS 1:19, 1:36, 1:47, 1:50–1:51, 2:4, 3:54–55, 4:25, and 4:32–34).

In essence, these sutras tell us that when we commit ourselves to the methodical practice of yoga sadhana we begin to see the deeper causes of the roaming tendencies of our mind. We realize that, while living in the world of primordial prakriti, we have created our own little world made of our likes and dislikes, attachments and aversions, fears and temptations, and have unwittingly become prisoners of our own creation.

Through yoga sadhana we discover the brighter and self-revealing part of ourselves. As our practice unfolds, both the binding forces of the subtle impressions deposited in our mind and the actions propelled by them become weaker. We become stronger in direct proportion to our mastery over our mind and samskaras. Eventually, we reach the point in our inner quest where the charms and temptations of sensory objects and the subtle impressions that feed them have little or no effect on us. Sutra 2:4 tells us that at this point our samskaras are *tanu*, attenuated. For the most part, we are free from avidya, asmita, raga, dvesha, and abhinivesha. Our mind is clear and we see our own inner luminosity.

As this stage matures, our samskaras become *prasupta*, dormant. Now we are free from all samskaras, including avidya. The purity of our mind is equal to the purity of our inner being, which is supreme consciousness. Our discerning power is unshakeable. We are still under the influence of the fully mature karmas fueling our physical existence, but at the spiritual level we are *jivan-mukta,* free from further karmic consequences. The karmas fueling our physical existence evaporate when we die (YS 2:10) and are absorbed into primordial prakriti without a trace of samskaras. The intrinsic prakriti of Ishvara becomes our locus and we reside there as *videha* or *prakritilaya* (YS 1:19). Videhas and prakritilayas are not established in the prakriti made of their samskaras but in their essential nature, which is *chiti shakti,* the intrinsic power of Ishvara. The rest of us are ordinary souls, and the karmashaya composed of our samskaras remains our locus after death.

The forces of sattva, rajas, and tamas manifest differently in these extraordinary souls than they do in us. These two modes of manifestation are known as *tulya jatiya* and *atulya jatiya. Tulya jatiya* means "manifestation mirroring its cause," and *atulya jatiya* means "manifestation somewhat dissimilar from its cause." Tulya jatiya manifestation occurs in the case of extraordinary souls—videhas and prakritilayas—while atulya jatiya manifestation applies to the rest of us.

Understanding the force behind these two modes of manifestation requires deeper analysis. Let us start with extraordinary souls and examine how the forces of sattva, rajas, and tamas manifest for them as they begin their world-bound journey. These souls have already completed their spiritual quest—they have reached a state where their kleshas, karmas, and karmashayas are so purified that no trace of samskaras remains. Their personal prakriti has been nullified. Their absolutely pure mind is no longer a mind in any worldly sense. Using this supremely purified mind as a locus, these souls dissolve into Ishvara's prakriti.

As sutra 4:32 tells us, such yogis are *kritartha,* souls whose purpose for being in the world has been fulfilled. In their case, sattva, rajas, and tamas, the intrinsic forces of prakriti, do not follow the ordinary laws of nature, which hold that cause and effect must remain connected to each other in a linear fashion. Manifestation is linear by definition—non-linear manifestation is outside the domain of the phenomenal world. As sutras 4:32–4:34 tell us, in the final stage of samadhi, extraordinary souls transcend the linearity of time, space, and the law of cause and effect. At death, they are absorbed into Ishvara's transcendental prakriti and emerge at the dawn of creation, bypassing ordinary laws of time, space, and the phenomenon of cause and effect. Sattva, rajas, and tamas do not interact with each other the way they interact in the case of ordinary souls. As Vyasa tells us in sutra 2:27, videhas and prakritilayas have attained *chitta vimukti,* freedom from the mind itself. They are *amala,* devoid of impurities. They are *kevali,* just that. And they are *svarupa matra jyoti,* the light of their own essence. Because they no longer have asmita, their essence is Ishvara itself. Their return to the world is as unique as they are.

Echoing the experiences of the long line of sages, Vyasa describes how videha and prakritilaya yogis manifest at *pradhana vela,* the dawn of creation. The dawn of creation is one of the most intriguing concepts in the spiritual literature of India. The word for dawn in Sanskrit is *prabhata,* "the phenomenon of unique illumination." Just as dawn in our familiar world illumines the horizon before the sun appears, videhas and prakritilayas illuminate the horizon of *pradhana,* primordial prakriti, before the phenomenal world appears. They are inseparable from Ishvara's self-nature. The instant Ishvara becomes aware of his intention to bring about creation, these unique souls are also aware of it and emerge instantly.

The scriptures are full of stories of sages who emerged from the mind of Ishvara. Because time has not yet come into the view of consciousness at the point of their emergence, these souls are called primordial sages. Another name for them is *sadyojata,* "born instantly." As accomplished yogis in the previous creation, they were absorbed in *jyotishmati*, divine light. When they reappear at the dawn of the next cycle of creation, they reacquire a body of divine light. In this body, they shine on the horizon of Ishvara's consciousness. Tulya jatiya, the manifestation mirroring its cause, applies to this category of souls.

Here, in sutra 2:18, Vyasa explains how sattva, rajas, and tamas operate to form a body fit for these special souls. As described in sutras 4:32 and 4:33, in the case of these unique souls there is no interaction among the three gunas because the intrinsic forces of primordial prakriti are in a state of perfect equilibrium. At the dawn of creation, driven by the sheer intention of Ishvara, one of these forces—sattva for example—comes forward to form the body of these special souls. Because the two other forces—rajas and tamas—are intrinsically present, they come forward to support the force of sattva, but for all intents and purposes, sattva alone manifests. It is in this context the scriptures tell us the body of Vishnu, for example, is made of pure sattva, as are the bodies of other great souls, such as Sanaka, Sanandana, Sanatkumara, Sanatsujata, and the seven sages.

This unique category of creation opens the door to understanding the most esoteric dimension of spiritual experience. According to the science of tantra, the manifestation of mantras belongs to this unique category. Mantras are living beings, and like the great sages, they emerge directly from the primordial prakriti of Ishvara. The body of the high-caliber sages is made of the subtle essence of light, whereas the body of mantra is made of the subtle essence of sound. The subtle essence of sound is pure and sattvic. The forces of rajas and tamas accompany sattva, but are relegated to the background. Mantras are as illuminating as the primordial sages and as immortal and beginningless. The forces of the phenomenal world have no power to influence mantras. Neither the seeing power of the sages nor the revealing power of the mantras can be obstructed. Because mantras are free from avidya, asmita, raga, dvesha, and abhinivesha, these afflictions melt away in their presence. As ordinary souls, we have no capacity to see these afflictions but we experience them; similarly, we have no capacity to see the mantras, but if they have made our mind their abode we experience them.

The manifestation of the primordial sages and mantras is tulya jatiya because their defining attributes (*jatiya*) are similar (*tulya*) to their origin—Ishvara's prakriti. Their body is as pervasive as Ishvara's body. Their knowledge is as limitless as Ishvara's knowledge. They are as untouched by karmas, karmashayas, and the five afflictions as Ishvara. Their virtues are as immaculate as Ishvara's and their divine effulgence is unobstructed. Their actions, like Ishvara's, are neither virtuous nor non-virtuous. During their manifestation, the forces of sattva, rajas, and tamas are not in a state of agitation. The sheer joy emerging from Ishvara's intention gently awakens them. The particular force needed to constitute the body of these unique beings takes the lead, supported by the other two forces.

How the three gunas relate to each other in the manifestation of these special beings is easy to understand if we recall how these forces function when a yogi reaches the highest state of samadhi. As sutra 4:32 tells us, in the highest state of samadhi the linear transformation of the attributes of prakriti comes to an end. In this state of absolute equanimity the forces of sattva, rajas, and tamas flow peacefully and do not commingle. For example, the flow of sattva is not influenced by the flow of rajas and tamas. When these high-caliber yogis re-emerge from primordial prakriti at the dawn of a new creation, the forces of sattva, rajas, and tamas function exactly as they functioned when the yogi was established in samadhi. The same purity of sattva, rajas, and tamas that characterizes samadhi characterizes their manifestation. Their manifest form is tulya, identical to their unmanifest form, and the manifestation of such beings is called *tulya jatiya.*

Those who are unfamiliar with the divine dimension of the gunas often associate sattva with spirituality and denigrate rajas and tamas. According to the sages, this error arises from ignorance. Ishvara's prakriti is as divine as Ishvara. The *Bhagavad Gita* calls it *daivi prakriti* as opposed to *manushi,* our terrestrial prakriti (BG 9:13). In the realm of primordial prakriti, all three forces—sattva, rajas, and tamas—are equally divine. That is why in tantric mythology, the goddess Sarasvati is equated with sattva, the goddess Lakshmi with rajas, and the goddess Kali with tamas. Vishnu's body is composed of sattva, whereas the bodies of Brahma and Shiva are composed of rajas and tamas, respectively.

At the dawn of creation, driven by divine will, an extraordinary soul may assume a body primarily composed of rajas or tamas. The primordial snakes, such as Vasuki, Shesha, and Karkotaka, are as pure and divine as their origin—Ishvara's prakriti—even though their bodies are primarily composed of rajas. Similarly, the prakriti of the primordial *daityas* (translated as "demon," for lack of an appropriate English word), such as Madhu, Kaitabha, and Vrishaparva, is as pure as Ishvara's prakriti, even though their bodies are principally composed of tamas. For this reason, scriptures refer to these beings as *divya naga*, celestial snakes, and *divya daitya*, celestial demons. Due to the lack of interaction between the intrinsic forces of nature, they carry an unyielding personality. A sattvic being of this stature cannot stop emitting sattvic energy. Similarly, extraordinary souls who primarily use rajasic or tamasic attributes of primordial prakriti as their locus emit rajasic or tamasic energy. The phenomenal world and the ordinary souls residing in it benefit from the sattvic, rajasic, and tamasic energies emitting from these special beings.

In our case, nature's forces—sattva, rajas, and tamas—interact with each other differently because they are contaminated by our samskaras. As we have seen, our samskaras are of a mixed nature. Even our most sattvic samskaras are invariably blended with a good measure of rajasic and tamasic impressions. As described in sutras 2:5–2:9, if left unchecked, our samskaras keep getting stronger. That is why samskaras churn our mind more violently during old age than they did when we were young. In Sankhya Yoga, this process is known as *guna-vaishamya-vimardana*, kneading the chaotic conditions of the gunas (*Sankhya Karika* 46). It accelerates our inner agitation—we become restless and frustrated. This internal churning and tossing drains the natural strength and acuity of our mind and senses. It also destroys the nine *tushtis,* satisfactions, and eight *siddhis,* extraordinary powers, which are our birthright. This process culminates in a state known as *ashakti,* disempowerment. This subject is discussed in detail in sutra 2:24.

Ashakti counteracts and eventually overpowers our life force, but before it does, samskaras storm our mind from every direction. The prospect of death causes panic, which destroys linear thinking. It breaks the link between the cortex and the limbic system and blocks the awareness of our self-identity. Finally, we drown in lack of awareness—we die. When we re-emerge, we pass through the same condition that clouded our mind when we were dying. There is the same churning and tossing of our samskaras, the same kneading of the chaotic conditions of the gunas. Unlike extraordinary souls who emerge on the horizon of Ishvara's prakriti, we emerge on the horizon of death. This is characterized by the relentless churning and tossing of our samskaras and gunas. Every samskara is supported in part and opposed in part by another samskara. We are as powerless as we were when we were dying. This is when the guiding grace of Ishvara descends. Prakriti breathes life into us. We rise above our disempowerment. Ishvara's guiding grace gently pulls us out of the event horizon of our death and helps us reclaim our memory and knowledge (BG 15:15). It transports us from the abstract world of our samskaras to the phenomenal world. *Atulya jatiya,* manifestation somewhat dissimilar from its cause, begins here.

In our journey from death to birth, we are brought into the phenomenal world at the time and place most conducive to finding the fulfillment and freedom we were seeking in previous lives. Conception unites us with the world of primordial prakriti. Although nature allows us to borrow the energetic and biophysical properties of our parents, our strong self-identity modifies these genetic properties. This is why the manifestation of our physical and psychological traits may be vastly different from that of our parents. All of us are primarily made of *tattvas,* the fundamental substances that have evolved from primordial prakriti, yet each of us is a distinct individual. Unlike extraordinary souls, we are more dissimilar from our origin than similar to it.

Atulya jatiya is always *shakti-bheda-anupati,* proportional to the power we have retained. The more disempowered we are, the more dissimilar we will be from our origin. As sutra 4:34 tells us, *chiti shakti,* unalloyed power of consciousness, is our essential nature. Because our avidya-driven samskaras contaminate and distort our essential power of consciousness, our personal prakriti—composed as it is of our samskaras—is quite different from Ishvara's prakriti.

In sutra 2:3, Vyasa describes a four-step process of waking from the slumber of death. As soon as the guiding grace of Ishvara casts its glance on us, the gunas—the intrinsic attributes of our personal prakriti—begin to pulsate and exert their influence on each other. This is the first step. The mutual interaction of these forces lays the foundation for change. This is the second step. In response, the currents of cause and effect are pulled together. This is the third step. Because the currents and crosscurrents of the forces of our prakriti are deeply entangled, their functions are heavily dependent on each other. In this environment of mutual dependency they bring our karmas to fruition. This is the fourth step. As sutra 2:13 tells us, karmic fructification determines *jati,* the general condition of our birth and the body into which we are born, *ayu,* our life span, and *bhoga,* the general course of our life experience. In regard to our jati, ayu, and bhoga, we are different from our parents.

We may die in a state of disempowerment, we may be conceived in a state of disempowerment, we may grow in the womb in a state of disempowerment, but as soon as we are born, much of this disempowerment is removed by nature. This is the beauty of a human birth. After we are born, our body, mind, senses, and nervous system develop in an astonishing way. Higher intelligence, which has been accompanying us throughout our long transmigration, fills us with a curiosity to discover the richness in which this world abounds, enabling us to absorb a vast amount of information relatively quickly.

The innate wisdom of our body and the immense power of our mind and senses are evidence that we are meant to understand the subtleties of the infinitely rich phenomenal world. We are meant to gather the tools and means to complete our unfinished task of finding fulfillment and freedom. Despite the limitations engendered by our samskaras, the primordial nature of Ishvara has given us the power to see and experience the phenomenal world correctly. Because everything in the universe is within the range of our understanding, the phenomenal world is described as *drishya,* perceivable, and we have the capacity to be *drastha*, the perceiver. The clearer our perception, the greater our chances of experiencing the fullness of our being. The world created by primordial nature is infinite, yet as Vyasa tells us in sutra 3:26, all of it is within the range of our comprehension. The human body, more precisely the *chakras*—the vortices of consciousness in the body—are the gateway to discovering the mystery of the universe and our life in it.

The vastness of Ishvara's prakriti, the vastness of the universe manifesting from it, and the extent to which we can comprehend this universe through perception, inference, or purely through intuition is the subject of the next sutra.

SUTRA 2:19

विशेषाविशेषलिङ्गमात्रालिङ्गानि गुणपर्वाणि ॥१९॥

viśeṣāviśeṣaliṅgamātrāliṅgāni guṇaparvāṇi ॥ 19 ॥

viśeṣa, specific; aviśeṣa, unspecific; *liṅgamātra*, barely describable; *aliṅgāni*, absolutely indescribable; *guṇaparvāṇi*, categories of gunas

The total range of the gunas is divided into four categories: specific, unspecific, barely describable, and absolutely indescribable.

This sutra serves as the foundation for yogic cosmology. Here Patanjali provides a succinct description of the range of primordial prakriti and the world manifesting from it. This manifestation has its source in the primordial prakriti of Ishvara and is known as *bhautika sarga,* creation consisting of matter and energy and the mental and sensory faculties of cognition. Another form of creation, *buddhi sarga,* evolves from our own mind. Because this second form of creation is composed of the personal cognitions and re-cognitions of our own mental material, it is also known as *pratyaya sarga,* creation consisting of cognitions. A student of yoga must take care not to conflate these two distinct forms of creation.

For centuries commentators and translators have used the terms *purusha* and *prakriti* somewhat loosely. This imprecision has caused confusion in discussions pertaining to yoga cosmology and eschatology. The confusion begins with the oversimplification of verse

21 of the *Sankhya Karika*: "Like a lame person and a blind person, purusha and prakriti unite. Attaining right understanding and liberation is the intention behind this union. This union is the cause of creation." A shallow interpretation of Sankhya philosophy and metaphysics has arisen from misreading this and similar passages.

According to this shallow interpretation, purusha and prakriti are both absolute and eternal and yet are completely different: purusha is intelligent and prakriti is unintelligent. Purusha is like a lame person and prakriti is like a blind person—they need each other's help to envision and execute a plan to extricate themselves from the cycle of creation, for, according to this interpretation, creation is full of sorrow. Thus purusha and prakriti unite with the intention of attaining freedom, and the very creation they are trying to avoid emerges from their union. Down through the centuries, scholars have mounted various arguments to justify this union as the cause both of creation and of freedom from creation, but none of these arguments stand up under reasoned scrutiny.

Yogis like Kapila, Patanjali, Vyasa, and other masters of the tradition offer a clear, crisp metaphysics and cosmology of yoga simply by defining the context in which the terms *purusha* and *prakriti* are used. As we will see, these two terms are used in two quite different contexts. There is a special purusha, and its prakriti is as special as that purusha. There is an ordinary purusha, and its prakriti is ordinary. Ishvara is a special purusha, and her prakriti is primordial prakriti. We are ordinary purushas and our samskaras are our prakriti. From the union of the special purusha and her prakriti, this beautiful and unimaginably vast universe ensues. From the union of ordinary purushas and their prakritis a personal world filled with afflictions manifests.

The "union" of the special purusha and its prakriti takes place outside the realm of time and space. It is not actually a union at all, for Ishvara's prakriti is inseparable from Ishvara. Like heat in fire and wetness in water, they are one. The analogy of a lame and a blind person does not apply to Ishvara and her prakriti. Ishvara is intelligent and intelligence is his prakriti. In the non-linear realm, the universe always exists as the essential nature of Ishvara. Through the sheer intention of Ishvara, the non-linear universe becomes linear. This is what is meant by "the manifestation of the universe from the union of special purusha and prakriti." Interpreting this union in finite terms is a profound mistake.

We are ordinary purushas. Our samskaras are our prakriti. As with Ishvara and her prakriti, union with our prakriti is also somewhat beginningless—it does not occur in the realm of time and space. Our samskaras are rooted in avidya and are constantly fed by it. Avidya is ignorance regarding our essential nature. We are ignorant about our ignorance. We do not know exactly when we became ignorant—thus practically speaking, our avidya is beginningless. Each time we die, the world made of our cognitions, along with our ignorance regarding ourselves, dissolves into the infinite prakriti of Ishvara.

As explained in the previous sutra, high-caliber souls—*videhas* and *prakritilayas*—dissolve into the intrinsic prakriti of Ishvara with full awareness, while ordinary souls dissolve into the same source without awareness. As detailed in sutra 2:24, avidya engenders twenty-eight *ashaktis,* twenty-eight forms of disempowerment. As a result, we sink into the slumber of death as a disempowered soul. Lying dormant in the layers of death, we have neither the capacity to see ourselves nor the capacity to move. Thus figuratively speaking, ordinary purushas and their prakritis are blind and lame. A unique world manifests from the union of these disempowered entities. Following the doctrine of *satkaryavada,* this world invariably contains all the elements of disempowerment lying dormant in these entities. Remember, the word *union* must not be taken literally, because in every respect we are intermingled with our prakriti. In fact, this intermingling is why we have fallen into the category of ordinary souls.

As disempowered souls, we have neither the capacity to know that we are dead nor the capacity to decide whether or not we should be born. The capacity to become aware of ourselves and our prakriti is granted to us through the sheer compassion and intention of Ishvara. This intention breathes new life into us—a degree of knowledge and memory returns. We become aware of our mental world, and a desire arises to see and experience our world vividly. The same compassion-driven intention plants us in the world that has evolved from Ishvara's primordial prakriti. From here we gather the materials necessary for the formation of our body and sense organs. Using these tools we experience the world of our samskaras, our unfulfilled desires, and our endless cravings. This is *pratyaya sarga*, the manifestation of our cognitions. It is not the subject of this sutra.

The subject of this sutra is *bhautika sarga*, the entire range of the universe manifesting from primordial prakriti. In this scheme of evolution there are twenty-four *tattvas. Tattva* is derived from *tat*, that. Throughout the spiritual literature of India, *tat* is used to indicate the ultimate reality. The Upanishads call this ultimate reality *brahman*. The *Bhagavad Gita* calls it *paramatman*. In the *Yoga Sutra*, Patajanli calls it *Ishvara.* Following the grammatical rules of Sanskrit, when combined with the suffix *tva*, the word *tattva* means "the essence of that." Primordial prakriti is the subtlest essence of "that," Ishvara. It is beyond our comprehension and thus indescribable. In the Sankhya scheme of the evolution of creation, primordial prakriti is the first and foremost tattva, the essence of Ishvara.

Because there is no English equivalent that will convey the entire meaning of *tattva*, it is usually translated as "element." But *tattva* is not "element" as understood in the fields of chemistry or physics. Rather, *tattva* conveys the powerful yogic doctrine that everything in the universe, beginning with the most subtle, indescribable, primordial prakriti all the way through the gross and tangible aspects of creation—such as earth and water—is a stage of the manifestation of Ishvara's essence. Every aspect of creation is divine and imbued with the power to dispel our primeval avidya. That is why in the previous sutra Patanjali states that everything in the world is meant to help us find lasting fulfillment and ultimate freedom.

Patanjali divides the twenty-four tattvas in the Sankhya scheme of evolution into four categories and lists them in order, from the grossest to the subtlest: *vishesha, avishesha, lingamatra,* and *alinga.*

The Four Broad Categories of Manifestation

Alinga

Primordial prakriti (beyond any point of reference)

Lingamatra (all-pervading subtle intelligence which can only be indicated)

Mahat/buddhi

Avishesha (6 "unspecific" tattvas)

Asmita

the pure sense of "I-am-ness"

5 tanmatras

the essence of sound, touch, form, taste, and smell

Vishesha (16 "specific" tattvas)

Manas

5 senses of cognition, which enable us to:

smell, taste, see, touch, and hear

5 senses of action, which enable us to:

grasp, move, speak, procreate, and eliminate

5 distinct categories of elements:

earth, water, fire, air, and space

Vishesha, "specific, unique, or distinct," is a technical term referring to a group of sixteen tattvas: the five distinct elements (earth, water, fire, air, and space); the five distinct powers of action (the power to grasp, move, speak, procreate, and eliminate); the five distinct sensory powers of cognition (the power to smell, taste, see, touch, and hear); and the power to think (the mind). These sixteen tattvas are vishesha, specific or unique, because they are the final stages of the creation manifesting from primordial prakriti. Nothing further evolves from them—they are the effect of more subtle tattvas but are not the cause of other tattvas. Any change or transformation we observe in them is actually a transformation in their *dharma,* attribute, their *lakshana,* sign, and their *avastha,* state—a subject elaborated on in sutra 3:13.

Furthermore, these sixteen tattvas are unique because they are infused with the powers of the *aghora, ghora,* and *ghora-ghora-tara* shaktis of Ishvara. As the *Shiva Sutra* states, "From the concentration of shaktis comes the birth of the body" (SS 1:19). These shaktis are the purest essence of Ishvara—they are Ishvara's prakriti. They breathe life into the distinct elements of earth, water, fire, air, and space; thus matter becomes animate and begins to pulsate. When these shaktis breathe life into our mind, the mind begins to sense its own existence and the existence of the unique properties of earth, water, fire, air, and space. The mind begins to feel its own inherent cravings and, in response, begins arranging the animate particles of the five elements to create limbs and sensory organs. Using these limbs and sensory organs, the mind attempts to explore the vast universe of primordial prakriti.

Avishesha, "unspecific," refers to a group of six tattvas: the five tanmatras and asmita. The five tanmatras are sound, touch, form, taste, and smell. They are far more subtle than what we understand of sound, touch, form, taste, and smell. They are *matra,* the pure and pristine potential shakti of *tat*, Ishvara. The aghora, ghora, and ghora-ghora-tara shaktis are in their unmanifest form in the five tanmatras. While they remain unmanifest, they do not serve the purpose of fulfillment and freedom for ordinary purushas, but as soon as these shaktis awaken, the five tanmatras are transformed into space, air, fire, water, and earth. In other words, the five tanmatras are the cause of their material counterparts.

The sixth unspecific tattva, asmita, is the pure sense of I-am-ness. In this pure state of I-am-ness, particularities pertaining to our self-awareness are not yet manifest. Unless these particularities manifest, asmita does not serve the purpose of fulfillment and freedom. As soon as the inherent particularities of the sense of I-am-ness awaken, the mind and the forces of the ten senses manifest. In other words, asmita is transformed into the mind and the senses.

The five tanmatras and asmita are the cause of the visheshas—the group of sixteen tattvas—but they are themselves effects of an even subtler tattva, known as *mahat tattva,* which, in Patanjali's terminology, is known as *lingamatra. Lingamatra* means "that which can be understood only through a sign." It is the subtlest aspect of the manifest form of unmanifest primordial prakriti. It is beyond the reach of our ordinary mind and senses, and so can be understood only through inference and scripture.

Two other terms used interchangeably describe the core content and dynamics of this subtle category of manifestation: *sattamatra* and *mahat. Sattamatra* is a composite of *satta* and *matra. Satta* means "existence," more precisely "the essence of *sat,* being"; *matra* means "only." As Vyasa explains, *lingamatra* is *atmanah sattamatram,* only the existence of *atma,* Ishvara. It is Ishvara's own field of awareness, which he identifies with himself. In other words, lingmatra is a field of unalloyed consciousness charged with Ishvara's self-identity. The second term, *mahat,* adds another perspective to the description of this level of manifestation. The literal meaning of *mahat* is "great." Nothing in the manifest world is greater than this reality. The pervasive nature of mahat tattva cannot be quantified. It is the first stage of manifestation emerging from Ishvara's prakriti. Scriptures describe this stage of manifestation with various terms: *mahat, buddhi, mati, prajna, samvitti, khyati, chiti, smriti, asuri, hari, hara,* and *hiranyagarbha* (Mathara's commentary on *Sankhya Karika* 22).

In the state of mahat, the primordial forces of sattva, rajas, and tamas are pulsating with Ishvara's intention of manifesting her *svabhava,* her own unmanifest self-nature. This intention makes the unknowable knowable. This is the point at which the perceiving power of the perceiver becomes somewhat perceptible; the indescribable becomes somewhat describable. The purity of the manifestation at this stage is equal to the purity of its source, Ishvara. Thus, according to yoga, mahat tattva is what is being indicated by the term *God.*

Describing the nature of mahat tattva, the Vedic sage Narayana proclaims his experience: "I know this *mahat purusha.* It is as luminous as the sun and is beyond darkness. One transcends death only after knowing him. There is no other path. Prajapati, the lord or father of ordinary beings, moves in the womb [of mahat tattva]. Upon being conceived in this womb, he manifests manifold. The highest-caliber yogis see the *yoni,* the origin of that purusha, completely. The entire world is established in him. He shines for all celestial beings. He is in the forefront of the gods. He is born before any of the gods. I bow to the brilliance of that pure essence of inner intelligence" (*Yajur Veda* 31:18–20).

In Indian mythology we read about many *prajapatis,* primordial fathers. These primordial fathers are sometimes said to manifest directly from Brahma, the creator. They are also said to assume the role of Brahma, and all of them are said to be *rishis,* seers. Furthermore, the scriptures that enumerate these prajapatis and rishis emphasize that they are not separate entities but are one and the same. This leaves us embroiled in an endless debate about whether the sages posit polytheism or monotheism.

According to Sankhya Yoga, videha and prakritilaya yogis are what are known by the terms *Prajapati, Brahma,* and *deva*. They have transcended the entire realm of avidya and asmita. Thus they are not individual beings in any sense of the word. They have transcended time and space; therefore, the idea that they are born from someone or something is null and void. They are established in themselves. They emerge from themselves, abide in themselves, and are reabsorbed in themselves. They are one with the prakriti of Ishvara. Because our experience of that prakriti can reach only as far as mahat tattva, from our standpoint (as we saw in the passage from the *Yajur Veda*), they *are* mahat tattva. Videha and prakritilaya yogis reside in the womb of mahat tattva. They are eternally aware of the essential nature of mahat tattva. While remaining above time, space, and the law of cause and effect, they rise from mahat tattva, illuminate the infinitely vast womb of mahat tattva, and thus facilitate the manifestation of the material world.

As the *Bhagavad Gita* tells us, mahat tattva is where the phenomenal world is conceived. Ordinary souls have a chance to be born only after the phenomenal world is conceived in mahat tattva. This is where clusters of individual souls are conceived and where they are reabsorbed at death (BG 9:4, 9:8, 8:19). Mahat tattva is as fecund as Ishvara's prakriti. As soon as ordinary souls are planted in it, so to speak, they become animate, begin to pulsate, and instantly become aware of their own existence—that is how asmita, the sense of I-am-ness, is born. Asmita is the essence of *jiva*, the individual soul. In fact, asmita *is* the individual soul. The innate tendency of asmita to explore and find itself results in identifying itself with the tanmatras. As we have seen, the tanmatras are extremely subtle and thus intangible; therefore, the inner intelligence of mahat tattva spontaneously guides the tanmatras to manifest as the five distinct elements of earth, water, fire, air, and space. That is how asmita and the five tanmatras evolve from mahat tattva. From this group of six, the remaining sixteen tattvas manifest.

Beyond mahat tattva lies purest prakriti. It is *alinga*, beyond any sign or symbol. Nothing is subtler than primordial prakriti (YS 1:45). It is Ishvara's own intrinsic self-awareness—her svabhava—and so is as intelligent as Ishvara. It is as primordial as Ishvara and as omniscient. Like Ishvara, prakriti is untouched by time and does not fit in any category. Strictly speaking, it is not even existent. In order to emphasize its "absolutely" absolute state of being, Vyasa coins another term, *nihsatta,* devoid of existence. What we understand by "existence" begins with mahat tattva, for which Vyasa coins the term *nihsatta-sattam,* the existence of non-existence. Thus, in the language of philosophers, primordial prakriti is indescribable. The describability of prakriti begins to emerge only at the level of mahat tattva. As Vyasa writes, the highest-caliber yogis place themselves in mahat tattva, and upon establishing themselves fully in this level of reality, they begin to comprehend prakriti (*alingam pradhanam pratiyanti*) and eventually become established in it. Becoming established in prakriti means dissolving into Ishvara's own essence.

To reiterate, prakriti and Ishvara are one and the same. The evolution of the phenomenal world refers to the world evolving from Ishvara's own essence. The terms *prakriti* and *Ishvara* refer to a reality beyond time and space and the law of cause and effect. The relationship between the "two" is *avinabhava,* one cannot be without the other. From different vantage points, these two can be described as the body and soul of each other (*Saundaryalahari* 34). From here evolves mahat tattva, the creative matrix of the universe. This evolution is as spontaneous and timeless as Ishvara's intention. Mahat tattva is as grand as Ishvara's intrinsic prakriti in every respect, and is infused with pure intelligence. Scriptures refer to this as *hiranyagarbha,* the golden womb. The Vedas call it *jatavedas,* the fire that knows everything about everything ever born. Puranic texts call it Brahma, Vishnu, or Shiva. Tantric texts call it *yoni,* the creative matrix.

The totality of existence, including all liberated and unliberated souls, rests in this undifferentiated field of intelligence. Fully enlightened, liberated souls know the mystery of this existence; unliberated souls do not. *Avishesha* (the group of six unspecific tattvas) and *vishesha* (the group of sixteen specific tattvas) manifest from mahat tattva for the sake of the infinite number of unliberated beings. The universe consisting of twenty-two tattvas and all liberated and unliberated beings springs from mahat tattva and returns to mahat tattva at the time of dissolution. For all intents and purposes, the intrinsic forces of prakriti—known as sattva, rajas, and tamas, or as aghora, ghora, and ghora-ghora-tara—pulsate in the realm of mahat tattva, whereas in Ishvara's intrinsic prakriti, these forces remain in their absolutely equanimous state.

The world made of twenty-two tattvas is infused with everything that exists in mahat tattva. As Vyasa explains, the highest-caliber souls, such as videha and prakritilaya yogis, use their body, mind, and senses and the world around them to experience *vivriddhi-kashtha,* the furthest frontier of divine grandeur. Ordinary souls are also seeking the same divine grandeur, but without knowing what they are seeking. Videha and prakritilaya yogis see and embrace this grandeur; ordinary souls do not. Why these high-caliber souls see this truth and ordinary souls do not is the subject of the next sutra.

SUTRA 2:20

द्रष्टा दृशिमात्रः शुद्धोऽपि प्रत्ययानुपश्यः ॥२०॥

draṣṭā dṛśimātraḥ śuddho'pi pratyayānupaśyaḥ ॥ 20 ॥

draṣṭā, seer; *dṛśimātraḥ*, the sheer power of seeing; *śuddhaḥ*, pure; *api*, even; *pratyayānupaśyaḥ*, one who sees only what is being shown by buddhi

The sheer power of seeing is the seer. It is pure, and yet it sees only what the mind shows it.

Each of us is an extension of Ishvara. We are as pure, self-luminous, and joyful as Ishvara; our power of seeing is as boundless as Ishvara's seeing power. Yet in spite of this, we rarely experience our connection with Ishvara. We are far removed from Ishvara's purity and are more acutely aware of pain than joy. In this sutra, Patanjali and Vyasa explain why we are not able to see who we are.

Ishvara is *svarupa pratishtha,* established in his essential nature. Her power of seeing is not hindered nor is her purity compromised. Ishvara's luminosity is unobstructed and its joy untainted. Although we are extensions of Ishvara, we are not svarupa pratishtha—rather we are *buddhi pratishtha,* established in our buddhi. Our power of seeing is hindered by our samskaras—our likes, dislikes, urges, and habits. Our purity is compromised by the five afflictions—avidya, asmita, raga, dvesha, and abhinivesha. Our luminosity is obstructed by the darkness of ignorance, and our joy is tainted by pain and sorrow.

Buddhi is the purest and sharpest of our mental faculties. It is *mahat tattva* in miniature. Just as mahat tattva gives definition to the indefinable—Ishvara and her intrinsic prakriti—buddhi gives definition to our indefinable essence. Just as the entire phenomenal world manifests from mahat tattva, the world stored in our karmashaya manifests from our buddhi. However, there is a vast difference between how mahat tattva relates to Ishvara and how buddhi relates to our essential self. This difference explains why Ishvara and high-caliber souls absorbed in Ishvara's intrinsic prakriti see the entire truth but we do not.

The purity of mahat tattva is identical to the purity of Ishvara; thus mahat tattva is fully illuminated by the luminosity of Ishvara's intrinsic prakriti. The purity of our buddhi, however, is not identical to our essence. Our buddhi's purity is contaminated by the long-cherished samskaras embedded in it and so is not fully illumined by our inner luminosity. Furthermore, our partially illuminated buddhi is constantly influencing our core being. Ishvara identifies with mahat tattva with full awareness and remains unaffected by this identification, while we identify with our buddhi without awareness and are affected by this identification.

Ishvara is not dependent on mental faculties to comprehend itself and mahat tattva, but we are completely dependent on our mental faculties to comprehend both ourselves and our buddhi. Because our buddhi is contaminated by its constituent samskaras, the comprehension it brings is invariably flawed.

Even when Ishvara descends into the fecund mahat tattva, he retains self-mastery. Our core being, on the other hand, does not descend into our buddhi; rather, we are united with our buddhi by the infallible intention of Ishvara and do not retain mastery over ourselves. The infinitely vast field of mahat tattva is infused with Ishvara, but Ishvara is not limited by mahat tattva. When we are united with buddhi, we become limited by it. Mahat tattva does not limit the seeing power of Ishvara—Ishvara's omniscience is forever unsurpassed—but as soon as we are united with buddhi, our omniscience evaporates. Figuratively speaking, we become blind. We see only what buddhi shows us. We experience only what buddhi allows us to experience. This is the condition of an ordinary soul.

Vyasa calls an ordinary soul *buddhi pratisamvedi,* the knower who knows what flashes on the screen of buddhi. He also tells us that this ordinary purusha is neither *sarupa,* similar to, nor *virupa,* dissimilar from, buddhi. Our strong identification with buddhi and our inability to see ourselves without its aid forces us to experience ourselves and our buddhi as one, even though intuitively we know we are pure consciousness. Intuition tells us that buddhi is a field of cognitions—we identify ourselves with our cognitions and the field that contains them. Even when we become aware of our self-existence, this awareness is experienced as a mental cognition. Thus the subject is itself experienced as an object. Furthermore, this cognitive experience remains in the forefront of our consciousness only as long as it lingers on the screen of our buddhi. As a result, we experience the constancy of our consciousness as an ever-fleeting stream of cognitions.

Whenever the stream of cognitions pertaining to our self-awareness is disrupted and the gap between two cognitions occupies our mind, we feel lost and empty. We feel a powerful urge to re-collect ourselves. Our karmic impressions create an atmosphere that impels us to retrieve our past self-identity, and the irresistible power of avidya superimposes this identity on our core being. This is how asmita is born. We become *jiva,* an individual soul with limited knowledge, limited self-identity, limited capacity, and limited goals and objectives. We have no access to our pure being. We persistently identify ourselves with endless pure and impure constituents of our individuality. We are caught between light and darkness, freedom and bondage, the desire to live in this world and the desire to extricate ourselves from it. This state of wanting and not wanting breeds confusion. Overcoming this confusion becomes our principal mission.

Life in the phenomenal world provides us with an opportunity to reflect on our true nature and discover the root cause of our confusion. A mind infused with the power of linear thinking enables us to trace our confusion back to its subtle cause. It gives us the ability to clearly see the connection between our current actions and our samskaras. The senses help us put our knowledge into action. The body gives the senses tangibility, while the phenomenal world provides an opportunity for our body, mind, and senses to once again attend to our unfulfilled desires. The power of discernment intrinsic to our most refined mental faculty—buddhi—helps us decide whether to keep running on the track of our desires or to renounce them once and for all. In other words, *buddhi tattva* ultimately determines the fate of ordinary souls. To emphasize this, Patanjali introduces the next sutra.

SUTRA 2:21

तदर्थ एव दृश्यस्यात्मा ॥२१॥

tadartha eva dṛśyasyātmā ॥ 21 ॥

tat, that; *artha*, purpose; *eva*, only; *dṛśyasya*, the objective world; *ātmā*, soul

The soul of the objective world [buddhi] is meant for purusha.

As we have seen, buddhi is *mahat tattva* in miniature. Buddhi is the direct evolute of primordial prakriti and is as subtle as mahat tattva. Its illuminative power is unmatched. Asmita (the faculty of self-identification), the five tanmatras (the subtle essence of sound, touch, form, taste, and smell), the five distinct elements (earth, water, fire, air, and space), the five sensory powers of cognition (the power to smell, taste, see, touch, and hear), the five powers of action (the power to grasp, move, speak, procreate, and eliminate), and the mind are all extensions of buddhi (YS 2:19). They are anchored in buddhi and are objects of buddhi's understanding. Discord between buddhi and any of these twenty-two tattvas nullifies their powers and privileges. These tattvas are alive, so to speak, as long as they are connected to buddhi. Thus buddhi is the soul of the objective world.

The guiding grace of Ishvara unites us with buddhi. The sole purpose of this union is purusha's *bhoga* and *apavarga*, fulfillment and freedom. Buddhi helps us accomplish this purpose by turning itself and the other twenty-two tattvas into our *karma bhumi*, the ground where we perform our actions. Buddhi manifests her intrinsic power of discernment to guide us on the path of action, enabling us to discern, decide, and act. We can see the difference between real and unreal, good and bad, right and wrong. We are also able to see the difference between the goal and the means of achieving it. This power of discernment is passed on to all the tattvas evolving from buddhi. That is why discerning power inheres in every aspect of the phenomenal world, including our body, mind, and senses. Buddhi has the power to connect itself with the power of discernment inherent in all insentient and sentient beings, which is how it guides us to acquire what is useful and discard what is not.

Buddhi is infused with eight powers: four have their source in Ishvara's prakriti, and four have their source in our prakriti. The four powers inherent in Ishvara's prakriti are *dharma,* pristine attributes of divinity; *jnana,* knowledge; *vairagya,* non-attachment; and *aishvarya,* omniscience, omnipresence, and omnipotence. The four powers arising from our prakriti are *adharma,* stained attributes of our samskaras; *ajnana,* distorted or limited knowledge; *avairagya,* lack of non-attachment; and *anaishvarya,* the limited capacity to know, to be, and to act. As described in the previous sutra, our core being and buddhi are completely intermingled. Due to our strong identification with our buddhi, we do not see the difference between our buddhi and our core being.

The ultimate goal of yoga sadhana is to identify our inherent powers and distinguish those that have their source in Ishvara's prakriti from those rooted in our prakriti. As we purify our mind we become increasingly aware of the subtle nuances of our inner world. As we become aware of this inner reality, the four powers rooted in our prakriti gradually lose their potency. The charms and temptations of the world fade in proportion to this awareness, and as they do, our experience of fulfillment and freedom no longer depends on worldly objects and achievements. In the final stage of yoga-born purity, buddhi—the innermost faculty of our mind—is so luminous that it is able both to see itself clearly and to see our core being reflecting in it. That is how as a combination of seer and seen, purusha and buddhi, we are guided to see the seer within. In the light of the seeing power of the seer, the afflicting contents of our karmashaya are rendered inert. Our samskaras become *dagdha-bija,* impressions that are like roasted seeds. At the dawn of this realization, we no longer see the phenomenal world as a source of bondage. We are *jivan-mukta,* free here and now.

The phenomenal world exists for our bhoga and apavarga. Once this purpose is achieved, does the phenomenal world continue to exist? The next sutra addresses this question.

SUTRA 2:22

कृतार्थं प्रति नष्टमप्यनष्टं तदन्यसाधारणत्वात्
॥२२॥

kṛtārthaṁ prati naṣṭamapyanaṣṭaṁ
tadanyasādhāraṇatvāt ॥ 22 ॥

kṛtārthaṁ, the one whose purpose is fulfilled; *prati*, toward; *naṣṭam*, destroyed; *api*, yet; *anaṣṭaṁ*, not destroyed; *tat*, that; *anya*, other; *sādhāraṇatvāt,* for the reason of being common

In relation to the one whose purpose is fulfilled, the objective world is destroyed, but in relation to others it is not destroyed, for the objective world is common to all purushas.

Here, as a follow-up to the previous sutra, Patanjali tells us that as soon as we see our core being, our purpose for being in the world is accomplished. We come to find fulfillment and freedom. We find fulfillment by discovering the desirable and undesirable qualities of the objects of our experiences and by immersing ourselves in them (*ishta-anishta-guna-svarupa-avadharanam avibhaga-apannam bhogah,* Vyasa on YS 2:18). We find freedom by discovering the essential nature of the experiencer (*bhotuh-svarupa-avadharanam apavargah*, Vyasa on YS 2:18). The phenomenal world provides the tools and means to accomplish this twofold purpose. A supremely purified mind (more precisely, buddhi) is the finest of these tools. Once this purpose is accomplished, the world in which we were born is withdrawn into *buddhi tattva,* and buddhi tattva is absorbed into *mahat tattva* (*Sankhya Karika* 36).

As an introduction to sutra 2:22, Vyasa makes an emphatic statement in the previous sutra: "Once the purpose of *bhoga* and *apavarga* is accomplished, the objective world is no longer seen by purusha. Due to the destruction of its essence, the world is destroyed but it is definitely not destroyed." Before the dawn of discerning knowledge, we see the objective world through the lens of our samskaras—our likes, dislikes, hopes, and fears. We project our samskaric coloring on worldly objects and experiences. When yoga-born purity takes effect and we begin to see things as they really are, we begin to see the desirable and undesirable qualities of our experiences accurately. We realize that immersion in an experience is what gives us a sense of fulfillment—objects themselves are neutral.

Before this realization, there was a subject-object relationship between the phenomenal world and us. Every object appeared to have a consumable quality (*karma-rupatam apannam*, Vyasa on YS 2:21). According to our unenlightened mind, this apparent consumable quality is *svarupa,* the essential property of worldly objects. At the dawn of discernment, this so-called essential property of worldly objects vanishes. This frees us from sensory cravings. It is in this sense that the world and worldly objects are said to be destroyed. In reality, the phenomenal world remains.

In this sutra, Patanjali tells us the phenomenal world, which no longer serves any purpose for an accomplished yogi, continues to serve the purpose of bhoga and apavarga for others. The relationship between our core being and our mind is beginningless. This union has created a unique world for each of us. From the standpoint of enlightened masters, we are prisoners of our unique world. We can extricate ourselves from this prison by using the powers and privileges inherent in the phenomenal world and, most important, those inherent in our own mind. How we accomplish this is the subject of the next sutra.

SUTRA 2:23

स्वस्वामिशक्त्योः स्वरूपोपलब्धिहेतुः संयोगः ॥२३॥

svasvāmiśaktyoḥ svarūpopalabdhihetuḥ saṁyogaḥ ॥ 23 ॥

sva, one's own; *svāmi*, Ishvara; *śaktyoḥ*, power; *svarūpa*, one's essential nature; *upalabdhi*, achievement; *hetuḥ*, means; *saṁyogaḥ*, union

The union of our shakti and the shakti of Ishvara is the means of experiencing our essential nature.

As sutras 2:20 and 2:21 tell us, the sheer power of seeing itself is the seer, and further, we are that seeing power. We are extensions of Ishvara; at the core we are as pure as Ishvara. Yet at this stage in our evolution, we are not able to experience our essential nature. We have no awareness of our pure and pervasive intelligence. We are so heavily dependent on our mind that we are able to see and experience only what our mind shows us. We are able to comprehend the depth of our own being and the vastness of the phenomenal world only in proportion to the purity and intuitive ability of our mind.

The mind lies at the center of our personal world. It is an extension of *mahat tattva*, an immense field of intelligence pulsating with creativity. The mind, which is as pure and luminous as mahat tattva, is a gift from primordial prakriti. The mind is designed to unveil its own essential nature as well as the essential nature of pure consciousness, but it has lost much of its self-revealing capacity because it has become cluttered by innumerable samskaras. In this sutra, Patanjali tells us how to reclaim the mind's self-revealing capacity and thus become established in our essential nature.

Three terms in this sutra are highly significant: *sva shakti, svami shakti,* and *svarupa.* At first glance, the meaning of these terms appears simple. *Sva shakti* means "the power of our mind and the world associated with it." *Svami shakti* means "the power of Ishvara and the world associated with her." *Svarupa* means "one's own essential nature." From this we can conclude that the meaning of the sutra is: "From the union of the power of our mind and the power of Ishvara we attain the knowledge pertaining to our essential nature." According to the tradition, however, this sutra is more profound than what is conveyed by this literal translation. A yogi aspiring to attain the highest goal of life must pay close attention to the deeper meaning.

Attaining knowledge of our essential nature (*svarupa upalabdhi*) and becoming established in it (*svarupa pratishtha*) are the reason we are born. The manifest world contains the tools and means we need to find life's purpose. As a faculty of discernment, our mind is a direct extension of the self-luminous creative field of intelligence. Originally, the illuminative quality of our mind was identical to the illuminative quality of pure consciousness, but in the process of our world-bound journey it has accumulated layers of karmic dust. As a result, the mind fails to illuminate itself and the phenomenal world. It fails to reveal either its own nature or the nature of the world inside and outside us. The goal of yoga sadhana is to remove the layers of dust so the revealing power of the mind can shine forth.

In yogic literature, the mind is described as a self-shining gem (YS 1:41). Elaborating on the pristine nature of the mind and its relationship to the supreme being, Shankaracharya writes, "In the middle of the ocean of ambrosia lies an island of gems with a garden of celestial trees. In the center of the garden is the palace of wish-fulfilling gems. In the courtyards of this palace are special gardens of plants pulsating with their inherent life force. In the innermost chamber of the palace, consciousness resides on a throne of its own intrinsic shakti. Fortunate are those who identify and embrace this divinity as a wave of consciousness and joy" (paraphrased from *Saundaryalahari* 8).

The mind is the palace of our core being. It is made of wish-fulfilling gems, for it has the capacity to help us find life's purpose—lasting fulfillment and freedom. The space inside our mind pulsates with *prana shakti,* the life force. The innermost chamber of our mind is the home of the divinity we are seeking. *Chit,* consciousness, and *ananda,* joy, are intrinsic to this divinity. At its core, our mind is lit by the luminosity of divinity. Dispersing pure awareness and joy is the defining characteristic of our mind. In yogic literature, this defining characteristic is known as *buddhi sattva.*

Buddhi sattva, the essence of buddhi, refers to the sattvic quality of primordial prakriti. Illumination is its fundamental quality—it is the self-revealing shakti of Ishvara in each of us. All of us are born with buddhi sattva; thus, in essence, each of us is a *bodhisattva,* a soul on the way to becoming Buddha. In this sutra, Patanjali explains what is preventing us from recognizing the illuminating quality of our buddhi sattva and, further, how to remove those obstacles and recognize our true essence.

At this stage in our evolution, we have become oblivious of the properties of our mind. As soon as we are born, we develop a strong sense of self-identity. In yogic terminology, this self-identity is *sva*; literally, "my." The power that engenders the sense of "my" is known as *sva shakti.* It is a unique power of the mind that claims ownership of itself. Under the influence of this shakti, the mind declares its independence from Ishvara—it rejects its association with Ishvara, along with Ishvara's guiding and nurturing grace, and begins to build its own personal empire. It attempts to own anything that happens to come into its view, beginning with the mind itself. Then it sees the body and claims ownership of that. It also claims ownership of all mental contents, and thus becomes the proprietor of numberless strands of samskaras. In this way, the mind creates a world parallel to the world created by Ishvara's primordial prakriti.

We are so engaged in attending and nurturing our personal world that we have totally forgotten Ishvara's intrinsic shakti, even though it fills the entire phenomenal world, including our own body, mind, and soul. It never occurs to us that we—as a mind or as a soul or as a combination of the two—have no capacity to create a body, a mind, or a soul. The fundamental elements of matter are the creation of Ishvara's prakriti. Sensory capacities and sensory organs evolve from the primordial pool of Ishvara's prakriti, yet in our ignorance we claim to be the owners of the world it has created. According to this sutra, this is how we have created a mind that is fundamentally flawed. Our dependence on this flawed mind is the cause of our lost identity and the source of our endless sorrow. To reclaim our pristine identity, we must repair this fundamental flaw. Patanjali tells us we accomplish this by uniting our *sva shakti,* the power of our mind, with *svami shakti,* the power of Ishvara.

The secret of uniting our mind and its powers with Ishvara is locked in the word *svami* itself. *Svami* is loosely translated as "master, lord, possessor." Following two different formulas of

Sanskrit grammar, *svami* has different meanings. The first is "one in whom *sva,* the phenomenal world including ourselves—our body, mind, senses, and all our strengths and weaknesses—exists" (*sva asti asmin iti svami*). The second meaning is "one who resides in every nook and cranny of *sva,* the phenomenal world" (*svasmin vasati iti svami*). Following the second formula, *svami* also means "one who resides in oneself." In this sutra, *svami* conveys all three meanings simultaneously.

Because we have fallen into the trap of our flawed mind, we do not know who our true creator, provider, guide, and protector is (*Bhagavad Gita* 7:13). We do not remember who initiated the *spanda,* pulsation, when we—along with our mind, senses, karmas, and karmashaya—were lying dormant in the dense darkness of death. Who planted the seed of life in the soil of death? Who incubated us? Who guided us to crack through the stiff shell of *asat,* nothingness, and emerge as a living being? Who infuses our mind with intuitive power, enabling us to comprehend ourselves? Who empowers our mind to feel and respond to the urges of hunger, thirst, sleep, and fear? Who enables us to concretize the abstract forces of time and space, break them into numberless segments, and arrange them in sequence? Who trains our organs to become acutely aware of sensory objects and pass these sensory experiences on to our brain? Who transforms our short-term memories into long-term memories and preserves them? Who enables us to retrieve select memories and keeps the rest out of our conscious awareness? Who runs our autonomic nervous system and visceral organs and keeps our mind free from numberless bio-behavioral details? In short, who raised the intelligent and perceptive being that we are? Patanjali's answer: svami shakti.

For untold ages we have been denying the shakti of our svami and have instead promoted the shakti of sva, the power of our mind. According to Patanjali, we do not need to reject the power of our mind. The mind is our most valuable asset and we must nurture it by connecting to its source. As soon as the mind recognizes the need for illuminating itself with the nurturing and self-revealing light of its creator, it drops its defenses. Then it sees itself correctly and sees the power of seeing seated in its own core. This experience is what Patanjali calls *svarupa upalabdhi,* attaining and becoming established in our essential nature.

At the practical level, the process of svarupa upalabdhi begins with cultivating the courage to see and confront our own flawed mind—and making a decision to trustfully surrender our little mind and its possessions to our svami, Ishvara, the lord of life. What is preventing us from cultivating this courage and deciding to surrender to Ishvara is the subject of the next sutra.

SUTRA 2:24

तस्य हेतुरविद्या ॥२४॥

tasya heturavidyā ॥ 24 ॥

tasya, of that; *hetuḥ*, cause; *avidyā*, ignorance

The cause of that [union] is ignorance.

In the ultimate analysis, our mind is not our mind but Ishvara's mind. *Buddhi sattva*, the mind's luminosity, is the luminosity of Ishvara—Ishvara's own intrinsic prakriti. Out of compassion Ishvara gave us a self-luminous mind, so that in its self-revealing light we can comprehend our essential nature as well as the nature of the objective world. Our claim to be the owner of "our" mind is the primal error. With this mistake, *sva buddhi*, "our" mind, is born (Vyasa on YS 2:23), and the extraordinary mind we received from Ishvara devolves into an ordinary mind.

In order to preserve its claim to its powers (*sva shakti*), the mind severs itself from the powers of Ishvara (*svami shakti*). It becomes weak and infirm—its capacity to discern and decide is heavily damaged. With the help of this debilitated mind we are trying to find our life's purpose, *bhoga* and *apavarga*. In the previous sutra, Patanjali tells us that the way to remedy this problem is to connect this weak, frail mind to its source, Ishvara, the fountainhead of all power and intelligence. In this sutra, Patanjali explains what prevents us from applying this remedy.

Vyasa explains that our primal error is propelled by avidya.

As soon as the self-luminous mind embraces avidya, it is transformed into *sva chitta* or *sva buddhi,* "our" mind. In effect, avidya is the seed that gives birth to our mind (*atha avidya svachittena saha niruddha sva-chittasya utpatti-bijam,* Vyasa on YS 2:23). The English equivalent of *avidya* is "ignorance." However, as we have seen in sutra 2:5, the mystery of avidya is as profound as the mystery of purusha and prakriti. In giving birth to our mind, avidya is as potent as primordial prakriti, which gives birth to *mahat tattva.* Avidya is as active in our mind as vidya is active in mahat tattva.

As a practical matter, avidya is the subtlest and most potent of all our samskaras—it is the samskara of our perverted understanding (*viparyaya jnana vasana*) and the root cause of all the afflictions. Asmita is central to this perverted understanding. Our sense of I-am-ness is so well developed that we see everything from the vantage point of our self-identity. We see soul, mind, senses, body, and the rest of the objective world only in relation to our self-identity. Thus we perceive them as "ours." From here, the three remaining afflictions—attachment, aversion, and fear of loss—evolve.

We spend our entire lives complying with the demands of avidya. We are constantly engaged in defending our self-identity. We are happy when we succeed in achieving the objects of our desires and unhappy when we fail. Likewise, we are happy when we succeed in getting rid of what we dislike and unhappy when we fail. Because we know nothing stays with us forever, we are always fearful. Our mistaken sense of self-identity, attachment, aversion, and fear of death are all continuously nourished by avidya, the subtlest and most powerful affliction.

When we analyze avidya's far-reaching destructive effect on our mind, we understand why removing avidya is absolutely crucial to finding life's purpose. As described earlier, our buddhi sattva, the essential attribute of our mind, is as pure, intelligent, and illuminating as mahat tattva, the first evolute of primordial prakriti. Buddhi, the discerning power of our mind, is flawless. It is given to us so we can see and assess the vast field of our mind and the numberless samskaras lying dormant in it. As soon as we are connected to this flawless mind, we become aware of the vast world of our mental contents. Most powerful among these contents is avidya itself. As soon as avidya emerges, we embrace it, ignoring the flawless mind that illuminated avidya and made it comprehensible. This embrace leads to the simultaneous emergence of sva buddhi, "our" mind, and rejection of the flawless mind.

With "our" mind, we attempt to accomplish an impossible task—exploring the world of our samskaras. Under the influence of avidya, we actively refuse to seek help from the pure, intelligent, and illuminating buddhi sattva, which pervades and permeates both our inner and external worlds. The tradition calls this phenomenon *buddhi vadha,* murder of the pure and pristine mind. We are left with "our" mind, a mind characterized by *ashakti,* disempowerment, which has twenty-eight manifestations. The *Sankhya Karika* divides them into three main categories: disempowerment of our mind and senses, disempowerment of our inner sense of fulfillment, and disempowerment of the powers unique to humans (SK 49).

The first category of ashakti is *ekadasha-indriya-vadha*, injury of the eleven senses. The eleven senses are the mind, the five senses of cognition, and the five senses of action (YS 2:19). With the murder of the pristine mind, our power of discernment is significantly eroded. Our self-understanding becomes dim and riddled with doubt. We lose a significant measure of trust and confidence in both ourselves and the objective world. We are no longer certain about our relationship with inner and outer reality. Disconnected from our source, we have neither the clarity nor the strength to face our samskaras—anything we know about ourselves and the subtle tendencies of our mind is contaminated with doubt.

In this atmosphere, we employ the mind to think, comprehend, decide, and act. Because our mind is plagued with doubt, we look to others to validate our thoughts and decisions. Furthermore, our mind now has only a limited capacity to illumine the broad range of the phenomenal world and so recognizes only one object at a time. It then works hard to string together a series of cognitions, and only after establishing a concomitant relationship between those cognitions does it arrive at a conclusion. Because its luminosity is contaminated and fragmented by the numberless samskaras contained in it, the chain of cognitions is also dimly lit and fragmented. As a result, our memory is significantly weakened. The weaker the memory, the harder it is to recall our experiences and learn from them.

By retrieving the experiences of the past stored in its own depths, the mind infuses the sense organs with its own power of cognition. In other words, the mind imparts its five distinct powers of cognition—smelling, tasting, seeing, touching, and hearing—to the corresponding organs. Similarly, the mind imparts the five distinct powers of action—grasping, moving, speaking, procreating, and eliminating—to the corresponding limbs and organs. Injury to the mind automatically affects the functions of our senses, because the mind is the master of our senses. Thus the dullness of our mind leads to a dulling of the senses. Experiences brought by dull senses are not fulfilling—they lead neither to fulfillment nor to freedom .

The second category of disempowerment is *tushti,* the deluded sense of satisfaction (SK 50). There are nine tushtis: *prakriti tushti, upadana tushti, kala tushti, bhagya tushti, arjana tushti, rakshana tushti, kshaya tushti, atripti tushti,* and *uparati tushti.* The first four belong to the internal realm, and the last five to the external realm.

The deluded internal satisfactions are extremely subtle. They cripple our ability to broaden the scope of our consciousness and force us to explore our grandeur solely within the confines of our disempowerment. We will briefly examine each one.

The first deluded internal satisfaction is *prakriti tushti,* our belief that we know prakriti—the building blocks of our body, mind, senses, and the objective world. Blinded by this deluded belief, we become rigid in our opinions. As a philosopher or a scientist, for example, we refuse to believe that the truth is more encompassing than all religious, philosophical, scientific, and metaphysical theories and discoveries combined. This misplaced belief is a symptom of our mental and intellectual disempowerment. A yogi under the influence of prakriti tushti believes that because he has studied and understood the difference between purusha and prakriti, he is no longer in bondage—he believes he is free. A scientist under the influence of prakriti tushti believes that because she has studied and understood the relationship between genes and diseases, she will conquer disease.

Prakriti tushti is a unique form of avidya—it blocks our vision of the infinite possibilities inherent in prakriti. With a mind shrouded by this veil, we conjure up a concept of the highest reality and then manufacture a relationship with it. Thus a Hindu and a Christian, for example, each have their own concept of higher reality and a way of establishing a relationship with it. Both aspire to experience higher reality in their own unique way, and both consider their unwavering faith to be a spiritual virtue. This engenders the idea of numberless gods and goddesses and sows the seeds of duality and difference.

Prakriti tushti evolves into *upadana tushti,* satisfaction associated with the external trappings of spirituality. Satisfaction derived from receiving a spiritual name, a special garment, or a mala are examples of upadana tushti. We know acquiring a peaceful, focused mind is a personal pursuit—no one else can purify our mind and turn it toward the center of consciousness, yet under the influence of avidya, we expect someone or something outside us to give us salvation. This expectation is a symptom of a disempowered mind.

The third deluded internal satisfaction is *kala tushti. Kala* means "time." Under the influence of this tushti, we fall into the grip of procrastination and inertia. We tell ourselves that time is a significant factor in any process of maturity—just as with time we become an adult, with time we will gain inner wisdom. We begin our quest halfheartedly, and when we do not succeed, we console ourselves by saying the time was not right. Attributing our success and failure to time, especially in relation to our spiritual journey, is a symptom of a disempowered mind.

The fourth and final deluded internal satisfaction is *bhagya tushti,* reliance on fate. We do not know what fate is, how fate walks into our life, and who governs and guides the forces of fate. We know that a seed sprouts only when we plant it and grows only when we tend it, but even so, we hope our inner growth will happen magically. "If I'm destined to be enlightened, providence will arrange the circumstances for enlightenment to dawn"—this idea is a symptom of a disempowered mind.

The five external tushtis—*arjana tushti, rakshana tushti, kshaya tushti, atripti tushti,* and *uparati tushti*—are self-fooling tendencies the mind uses to avoid engagement in worldly matters. The deep-rooted samskara of inaction convinces the mind to entertain thoughts such as: "Earning money and acquiring worldly resources causes pain. I'm happy with what I have." "Protecting what we have causes pain. I'm happy with what I lose and with whatever remains." "Following the law of nature, everything is subject to decay and destruction. I have no concern with what is preserved and what is destroyed." "Worldly objects and achievements are never enough. Therefore, I do not care what I have and what I lack." "The more involved we are in worldly affairs, the greater the sorrow. Therefore, I distance myself from the world."

Disconnected from its own inner brilliance, the mind cunningly convinces us there is no point in acquiring worldly resources (*arjana*) and protecting them (*rakshana*). It also convinces us that there is no point in being vigilant about preserving the resources we have acquired (*kshaya*). It convinces us that active engagement in worldly endeavors is a source of disappointment (*atripti*), and in order to find true fulfillment and freedom we must disengage from worldly activities (*uparati*).

Under the influence of these nine forms of pseudo-satisfaction, we commit ourselves to inertia and become passive and fatalistic. Yet there is an even more devastating effect on our evolution—the mental disempowerment that damages our *siddhis,* the powers and privileges unique to humans. These siddhis are *uha, shabda, adhyayana, dukha-vighata-traya, suhrit-prapti,* and *dana* (SK 51).

Uha means "knowledge without doubt, clear understanding, intuitive knowledge." It is the power of revelation—the fundamental force behind all human discovery. It has its source in mahat tattva, the pure and pristine manifestation of Ishvara's prakriti, and is therefore infinite. In our day-to-day life, it manifests in the form of discerning power. This is also the force behind our memory. As humans we have the privilege of harnessing this shakti and retracing our way back to the primordial being, Ishvara.

Shabda means "word." We are born with the capacity to give a form to sound, assign meaning to each segment of sound, and store both sound and its meaning in our memory. We have the capacity to communicate both sound and its meaning to others. We also have the capacity to give a visual form to each segment of sound and the meaning associated with it. This unique capacity has enabled us to develop written languages and preserve a vast range of memories pertaining to human experience.

Adhyayana means "study, analyze, and comprehend." We have the capacity to study, analyze, and comprehend an abstract idea whether it is spoken, written, or implied. We even have the capacity to decipher our own and others' intentions and predict the causes as well as the far-reaching effects of those intentions.

Dukha-vighata-traya means "elimination of threefold sorrow—physical, mental, and spiritual." We are born with the capacity to understand both the cause and the cure of all our physical, mental, and spiritual diseases. We have the capacity to discover the tools and means to overcome our sorrow.

Suhrit-prapti means "cultivating a good heart; finding friends." Our body, mind, and senses are designed to carry an enormous range of feelings and the samskaras associated with them. Our power of discernment and intuitive wisdom enables us to distinguish good thoughts and feelings from bad ones, and cultivate the good ones further to enrich the virtues of our heart. The same capacity enables us to see beyond the boundaries of our little world and share our goodness with others. This capacity also motivates us to pass our achievements on to future generations.

The last category of our innate siddhis is *dana,* "the ability to give." We have both the wisdom and the courage to share what lawfully belongs to us with others. We are designed to experience the joy of giving. This joy is the architect of human civilization, characterized by self-sacrifice and selflessness.

These extraordinary powers distinguish us from all other species. Because of these powers we are able to see the impediments to our quest far in advance and prepare ourselves to remove them long before they manifest. Because of these powers we are able to comprehend the invisible forces of nature and harness them to improve the quality of our life. With the decline of our inner luminosity, we lose these powers to a significant degree. The cause of this decline is avidya. Therefore, according to Patanjali and Vyasa, nothing is more important than the removal of avidya.

In summary, embracing avidya results in the birth of "our" mind. Under the influence of avidya, the mind rejects its connection with mahat tattva, the infinite pool of intelligence and creativity. Getting rid of our mind (*chitta nivritti*) and replacing it with a pure and pristine self-luminous mind is the goal of yoga sadhana. According to the previous sutra, this happens when we allow our mind to unite with the forces intrinsic to the inner being. As soon as our mind faces the luminosity of Ishvara, avidya melts away, leaving us with buddhi sattva, the pure essence of Ishvara's inner luminosity. This self-luminous field becomes the locus of our self-awareness. This realization is *svarupa upalabdhi* (YS 2:23). To be firmly established in this realization is *svarupa pratishtha* (YS 4:34).

The process leading to self-realization is simple—surrender our mind to Ishvara. Surrendering our messy mind and receiving a fresh, self-luminous mind sounds like an excellent bargain but, in practice, it is one we are reluctant to make. How to overcome this reluctance and acquire a mind fit for unveiling our essential nature is the subject of the next sutra.

SUTRA 2:25

तदभावात् संयोगाभावो हानं तद्दृशेः कैवल्यम् ॥२५॥

tadabhāvāt saṁyogābhāvo hānaṁ taddṛśeḥ kaivalyam ॥ 25 ॥

tat, that; *abhāvāt*, from absence; *saṁyogābhāvaḥ*, absence of union; *hānaṁ*, freedom; *tat*, that; *dṛśeḥ*, of the seeing power of the seer; *kaivalyam*, state of consciousness free from all conditioning

From the absence of that [avidya] comes the absence of mingling [of consciousness with "our" mind]. That is freedom, the absolute state of the power of seeing.

This sutra is a summary of the five preceding sutras. In sutra 2:20, Patanjali tells us that the sheer power of seeing is the seer, and we are that seer. At our core, we are pure. Even though unbounded luminosity and joy are intrinsic to us, we are unable to see ourselves and experience our inherent joy. We are heavily dependent on the mind—a mind conditioned by its samskaras. We see only what our mind shows us and experience only what our mind allows us to experience. Vyasa adds that, at this stage in our evolution, our mind and core being are so intermingled that they appear neither similar nor dissimilar—for all intents and purposes, they are one and the same. Our mental conditioning and the pain and sorrow arising from it are the pain and sorrow of our core being. As long as our mind and core being are intermingled, we have no access to our inner luminosity or to our intrinsic joy. In order to accomplish life's purpose, we must distinguish one from the other and become established in our essential nature. Birth gives us an opportunity to recognize the truth pertaining to our essential nature and the world of our mental conditioning.

In sutra 2:21, Patanjali tells us that the phenomenal world is meant for us. It is replete with the tools and means we need to accomplish our goal of self-realization. Our mind—more precisely our faculty of discernment—is the soul of the phenomenal world, for it is the embodiment of intuitive wisdom.

However, as Vyasa tells us in sutra 2:23, when our faculty of discernment embraces avidya, it is instantly transformed into an ordinary mind. Its divine attributes and, most important, *aishvarya*—our unrestricted capacity to discern, decide, and act—fade. This is why we are no longer able to comprehend life's purpose, and why we fail to use the abundant resources hidden in our body, mind, senses, and the world around us.

In sutra 2:23, Patanjali tells us that all we have to do to reclaim our self-luminous mind is unite the forces of our mind with the forces of inner divinity. But in sutra 2:24, he reminds us that, because our attachment to our ignorance makes us reluctant to let go of our familiar self-identity, we are unable to change. Letting go of our old, frail, dull mind and replacing it with a new, vibrant, and self-luminous mind has become a seemingly impossible task.

Here, in sutra 2:25, Patanjali delineates the steps leading to recognizing our core being—the seeing power of the seer—and releasing it from the tyranny of our avidya-driven mind.

We are amazing creatures. Our actions are always purpose-driven. Our purpose can be divided into two categories: avoidance of pain and acquisition of pleasure. Sutra 2:15 tells us that in the ultimate analysis, all experiences—including those that appear pleasant—are painful. As long as our mind is contaminated by likes and dislikes, fear and doubt, we are bound to experience pain. Getting rid of this contaminated mind (*chitta nivritti*) is the ultimate pain reliever. We acquired a contaminated mind by embracing avidya. As soon as we renounce avidya, mental contaminants evaporate.

In the absence of avidya, the inherent brilliance of our pure and discerning mind automatically comes to the fore. We begin to see ourselves as we are. We also see *buddhi sattva,* the pristine nature of our mind. The same mind that was once the source of bondage now becomes the source of freedom. This highly assertive clarity and comprehension arising from buddhi sattva is *viveka khyati.* In the light of viveka khyati, we are able to see that we are the seer, the seeing power itself. With the dawn of viveka khyati, the darkness of ignorance and our mental creations fed by ignorance vanish. We are established in our essential self. Our dependence on worldly objects and the experiences pertaining to them comes to an end. This is *kaivalya,* the experience of *chiti shakti,* the power of pure consciousness, which presides over primordial prakriti.

This highly assertive clarity and comprehension of our pure consciousness dawns through practice and contemplation. However, Patanjali is fully aware that, in most cases, this state of realization does not last long. We glimpse it, but it soon disappears. We vaguely remember how it feels to be in that state, but we do not know how to recapture it. Why we fall from this experience many times before becoming fully established in it is the subject of the next sutra.

SUTRA 2:26

विवेकख्यातिरविप्लवा हानोपायः ॥२६॥

vivekakhyātiraviplavā hānopāyaḥ ॥ 26 ॥

viveka-khyāti, dawning of discernment; *aviplavā,* unshakeable; *hānopāyaḥ,* the means of nullifying sorrow

Unshakeable discerning knowledge is the means of nullifying the misery resulting from the avidya-driven union of purusha and prakriti.

As we saw in sutra 2:4, afflictions exist in four states: *prasupta,* dormant; *tanu,* attenuated; *vicchinna,* disjointed; and *udara,* fully active. When the five afflictions—ignorance, false sense of self-identity, attachment, aversion, and fear of death—are fully active, the mind is dragged into a state of disturbance, distraction, confusion, and stupefaction. We lose the peaceful condition of our mind and have difficulty focusing. With the practice of meditation described in "Samadhi Pada" (particularly sutras 1:33–36), we minimize the effect of the afflictions and, consequently, calm the mind's churning tendencies, even though the initial stage of meditation does not destroy the subtle causes of disturbance and stupefaction. The inherent property of the object of meditation, coupled with the power of our intention, creates an illuminating and peaceful meditative atmosphere. As long as the mind stays in this atmosphere, it is free from disturbing, stupefying, and distracting tendencies and their subtle causes—the afflictions. But as soon as the meditative atmosphere fades, the mind is once again in the grip of its churning tendencies.

Every time we meditate, the mind is charged with illuminating, peaceful energy, and its ability to stay in that state increases. A meditative atmosphere leaves no room for the disturbing, stupefying, and distracting tendencies engendered by deep-rooted samskaras of afflictions. Sutra 2:4 defines this as *vicchinna*, the state in which the afflictions are disjointed. As long as afflicting tendencies do not become active, our mind is clear and assertive. It is illuminated by intuitive wisdom and able to see the seer reflecting on its pure and pristine screen. The mind has regained its *buddhi sattva,* its intrinsic power of discernment, and thus is confident that its understanding both of pure being and of the objective world is correct. But when the tsunami of mental tendencies originating from the vast field of afflictions sweeps away the illuminating and peaceful atmosphere of our meditation, the mind is once again awash in unsettling thoughts.

We become established in our essential nature only through steady practice and constant awareness of life's purpose. An occasional glimpse of our true self is not enough. It is only when our deeply rooted samskaras, fed by avidya, become *tanu,* attenuated, and, eventually, *prasupta,* completely nullified, that we reach the state of *kaivalya*, the realization of our absoluteness. The primordial seed of avidya is incinerated by *viveka khyati,* the illuminating power of discernment.

In the light of viveka khyati, we begin to see inner reality, ourselves, and the external world as they are. At this point, the idea that the phenomenal world is meant for our fulfillment and freedom is no longer merely an intellectual hypothesis. We see the world as a divine manifestation. We feel Ishvara's intrinsic powers—sattva, rajas, and tamas (also known as *aghora, ghora,* and *ghora-ghora-tara shaktis*)—manifesting in everything and everyone. We experience life as a gift and are grateful to the primordial prakriti of Ishvara, who gave us this gift. Our self-effort pertaining to yoga sadhana concludes with viveka khyati, the pure and pristine power of discernment. This brings us to the state of *videha* and *prakritilaya*. As long as we are alive we live as *jivan-mukta*, free here and now, and after death we reside in Ishvara's intrinsic prakriti—a state known as *svarupa pratishtha.*

How do we know that we have gained viveka khyati and that our mind is permanently lit by its self-luminous discerning power? That is the subject of the next sutra.

SUTRA 2:27

तस्य सप्तधा प्रान्तभूमिः प्रज्ञा ॥२७॥

tasya saptadhā prāntabhūmiḥ prajñā ॥ 27 ॥

tasya, his; *saptadhā*, sevenfold; *prāntabhūmiḥ*, furthest frontier; *prajñā*, revealing knowledge

His discerning knowledge has seven spheres; the furthest frontier is *prajna*.

In the context of this sutra, it is important to recall the concept of samadhi Patanjali introduced in "Samadhi Pada" (YS 1:17–18 and 1:42–51). He divided the range of samadhi into two main categories: *samprajnata* and *asamprajnata*. For the sake of simplicity, we translated *samprajnata samadhi* as "lower samadhi." In lower samadhi, we are fully aware of the object of meditation, the process of meditation, and ourselves as meditator; thus it is called *samprajnata,* samadhi with cognition. Samprajnata samadhi is further divided into four parts: *vitarka anugata, vichara anugata, ananda anugata,* and *asmita anugata.* These four levels of cognitive samadhi describe the gradual deepening of our mental absorption. Cognitive samadhi is also known as *sabija samadhi,* samadhi with seed, for in this state, although we are free from the roaming tendencies of our mind, extremely subtle and virtually untraceable mental impressions still exist. When these mental impressions vanish completely, we land in the state of consciousness known as *asamprajnata samadhi.*

Asamprajnata samadhi is loosely translated as "higher samadhi." In higher samadhi, we have transcended the field of cognition pertaining to the object of meditation, the process of meditation, and ourselves as meditator. It is a supracognitive state in which we are free, not only from the roaming tendencies of our mind, but also from the virtually untraceable mental impressions, which have vanished once and for all. That is why this state of samadhi is also known as *nirbija,* samadhi without seed.

Sutras 1:47–50 describe a mysterious transitional state between these two states of samadhi. In sutra 1:48, that state is described as *prajna,* the self-luminous field of consciousness filled with truth. This is the highest yogic achievement and the culmination of human endeavor. Here samadhi as a process comes to an end.

The experience gained in the state of prajna nullifies the effects of samskaras without creating samskaras of its own. It is the purest and highest state of inner illumination. Prajna is intrinsic to Ishvara's prakriti. When established in this state, we are established in Ishvara's prakriti. Our mind is no longer "our" mind—it is Ishvara's mind. Our soul is no longer "our" soul, for we have come to an unshakeable realization that our individuated consciousness is an extension of Ishvara. "Our" inherent joy is essentially the joy of Ishvara. The notion of "I" and "my" has dissolved. What lies beyond this point is not in the realm of mental comprehension. Furthermore, the state beyond this point does not lie in the domain of human endeavor. We reach this indescribable, unfathomable state only through divine grace. There we see ourselves through the eyes of Ishvara and experience ourselves through the heart of Ishvara.

Just as Patanjali divides the range of samadhi into two parts in chapter one, here he divides the range of prajna into two main levels. This division is based on how brilliantly prajna is illuminating the mind. The illuminative quality of the first level frees us from the operations of the mind and so is known as *karya vimukti,* freedom from mental operations. The illuminative quality of the second level frees us from the mind itself and is called *chitta vimukti.* The first level indicates that the veil of ignorance is becoming thinner, and the light of the inner being is becoming brighter. The second level indicates that the veil of ignorance has vanished, and the entire field of our mind is fully illumined by the light of the inner being.

The unfoldment of the first level of prajna—karya vimukti—is described in four stages. As discussed in the two previous sutras, the self-revealing knowledge of our *buddhi sattva* shines forth in direct proportion to the disappearance of the darkness of ignorance. Through consistent practice and contemplation, the veil of ignorance becomes thinner and eventually vanishes. Long before it disappears we are able to clearly see ourselves, our mind, and its contents. With the dawn of this self-revealing knowledge we see life as it is. We see the pervasive nature of sorrow. We become aware of an undeniable truth: every experience, including those that are pleasant, is inevitably accompanied by pain. We see that pleasure is short-lived and leaves us with a sense of dissatisfaction that compels us to repeat the cycle.

This realization is far more refined and profound than mere intellectual understanding. It requires no verification. We know our understanding of our body, mind, senses, and the objective world is correct (*parijnatam heyam*). There is nothing more to be known (*na asya punah parijneyam asti*). This realization enables us to perform our actions without expecting lasting fulfillment. We discharge our duties wisely and selflessly. Samskaras engendered by actions performed in this mental climate have no binding effect. This is the first stage of the dawning of prajna, self-revealing knowledge.

As prajna intensifies, we are able to see the causes propelling our current actions. Through our discerning mind we are able to observe how samskaras pulsate in the depths of our mind and how these pulsations lay the foundation for change. We are able to see how the currents of cause and effect are becoming connected and, ultimately, how our actions bear fruit. In the light of intense intuitive wisdom, when we pay attention to the internal functioning of our mind, we are able to trace the subtle process of karmic fruition.

After going through this process several times, we become confident in our understanding of the relationship between cause and effect—between our deeply ingrained subtle impressions and our current experiences. This direct realization weakens the potency of our samskaras. We are confident that the causes that churn our mind with afflicting thoughts have become attenuated (*kshina heya-hetavah*). We also know there is nothing else to be attenuated or destroyed (*na punah kshetavyam asti*). We are confident that the process of karmic purification is gaining momentum and no force can slow it down. This is the second stage of the dawning of karya vimukti.

In the third stage, we know our samskaras have lost their potency—they no longer have the power to churn our mind. We also know the power of *nirodha samadhi,* the process of the inward journey that serves as an antidote to the outward manifestation of our samskaras. We have confidence in our ongoing practice of nirodha samadhi and its infallible effect. This realization fills our mind and heart with unshakeable faith in our practice. We do our practice for its own sake.

Now comes the dawn of the fourth and final stage of karya vimukti. At this stage, we realize we have achieved *viveka khyati*, the power of discernment, and further, we know this achievement is unshakeable. We no longer have any desire to see the causes of our mental operations—we know they have been rendered impotent and we do not need to make any further effort to attenuate or destroy them. We are free from the anxiety of accepting or rejecting karmas that are currently manifesting. We are at peace. At this stage, trustful surrender becomes our nature. Both fortune and misfortune have lost their luster. Beyond this point, the second level of prajna—chitta vimukti—dawns.

This second level of prajna is characterized by the dissolution of "our" mind—a subject discussed in sutras 2:23 and 2:24. At this level, the mind is so pure that nothing is preventing the light of the inner being from penetrating it. The entire mind is lit by the luminosity of the inner being. In this light, our mind realizes that all samskaras, including the subtlest—avidya—have disappeared. By embracing avidya, the mind disconnected itself from its source. Now, as avidya vanishes, the realization dawns that the feeling of being separate from the inner being was a painful mistake. With this realization, the mind is spontaneously withdrawn into its source (*sva-karane pralayabhimukha*). Along with the mind, all the memories are also withdrawn into the source (*tena saha astam gachchhanti*).

This extremely subtle process matures into the second stage of chitta vimukti. This stage is characterized by a supremely refined mind and memory. As sutra 3:55 tells us, the purity of the mind is now identical to the purity of Ishvara. The mind is no longer "our" mind; it is buddhi sattva, the pure essence of *mahat tattva*, the first stage of manifestation in which indescribable absolute reality becomes somewhat describable. In this second stage of chitta vimukti, the supremely refined mind merges with mahat tattva. This merger is yoga, union.

To shed further light on this supremely refined mind, Patanjali, following the footsteps of previous masters, presents a third and final stage. Here the seeing power of the seer is so intense that the seer sees nothing other than itself. The totality of our being is transformed into the sheer seeing power of the seer (*svarupa-matra-jyotih*). For all intents and purposes, "our" mind ceases to exist and pure buddhi sattva (*amala*), the intrinsic essence of pure consciousness, alone (*kevali*) remains.

Commenting on this sutra, Vyasa makes a point of dismantling widespread confusion about yogis and their achievements. Long before Patanjali, and up to this day, poorly informed spiritual enthusiasts have been fantasizing about high-caliber yogis sitting in caves with their eyes closed, completely unconcerned with the outside world. Contrary to this stereotype, Vyasa calls the accomplished yogi *kushala,* one who is skillful. A yogi is skillful, for she knows the true nature of the world; the true nature of her body, mind, and senses; and the true nature of her core being. A yogi is free from all illusions, including the illusion of expecting more than what this world can offer. At the same time, a yogi is able to identify the wonderful gifts contained in the body, mind, and senses, as well as in the phenomenal world. Therefore, a yogi is able to discern, decide, and act in the light of her prajna. Because she is operating at the level of pure and penetrating wisdom of inner reality, she is confident about the appropriateness of her actions and their consequences.

While living in the world, a yogi is as active as—if not more active than—anyone else. The only difference is that the actions of an accomplished yogi are free from doubt and fear, whereas our actions are contaminated by them. An accomplished yogi is comfortable while performing actions and equally comfortable when refraining from action. A yogi's accomplishment is characterized by freedom, not by action or the absence of it.

However, both Patanjali and Vyasa also recognize that yogic accomplishment culminating in the highest level of prajna is a process. For some, this process is quick; for others, it is somewhat drawn out. In the following sutras, Patanjali delineates a system whereby regardless of where we stand today in our personal evolution, we can begin our journey and one day become master of ourselves.

SUTRA 2:28

योगाङ्गानुष्ठानादशुद्धिक्षये
ज्ञानदीप्तिराविवेकख्यातेः ॥२८॥

yogāṅgānuṣṭhānādaśuddhikṣaye
jñānadīptirāvivekakhyāteḥ ‖ 28 ‖

yogāṅga, the limbs of yoga; *anuṣṭhānāt,* from the practice; *aśuddhikṣaye*, at the destruction of impurities; *jñānadīptiḥ,* the shine of knowledge; *āvivekakhyāti*, domain of unshakeable discernment

The practice of the limbs of yoga destroys impurities; thereafter, knowledge continues to brighten all the way to *viveka khyati*, the domain of unshakeable discernment.

As explained in sutras 2:24–27, avidya is the root cause of sorrow. When avidya disappears, so does sorrow. The disappearance of avidya goes hand in hand with the appearance of *viveka khyati,* unshakeable discernment. Unshakeable discernment is characterized by *prajna,* intense self-revealing knowledge. In the light of prajna, we achieve *karya vimukti,* freedom from the consequences of our previous actions, and attain *chitta vimukti,* freedom from our old mind. Chitta vimukti is a state in which our mind is so transformed that its purity is identical to the purity of Ishvara. This highly purified mind is known as *buddhi sattva,* the pure essence of *mahat tattva.* In other words, our individual mind has merged into mahat tattva. This merger is yoga. A yogi who has reached this level of purity and union is *videha* or *prakritilaya*—terms equivalent to *bodhisattva* in the Pali language.

Reaching the highest level of purity accompanying viveka khyati is a process. It requires us to make an effort to cleanse our mind of its long-cherished samskaras. We need to get rid of our old mind—a mind filled with fear, aversion, attachment, distorted self-identity, ignorance, and the vast field of impressions fed and propelled by these afflictions. The body and mind are totally intertwined; both are nurtured and held together by the power of breath. Because nature has established an indestructible relationship between breath, body, and mind, the purification and transformation of the mind inevitably involves disciplines pertaining to the body and breath. In this sutra, Patanjali introduces a system for transforming ourselves on all three levels.

As described in sutra 2:1, tapas, svadhyaya, and Ishvara pranidhana constitute the heart and soul of yoga. Because, these three components enable us to shake off our inertia and empower us to put the lofty principles of yoga into action, Patanjali calls his system *kriya yoga*, yoga in action. In this sutra, he introduces the idea that, just as body and mind are the locus for our soul, yoga—which is composed of tapas, svadhyaya, and Ishvara pranidhana—also has a body as its locus. Just as our body consists of various limbs and organs, the body of yoga has its own components. The health of our body and its ability to serve the purpose of the soul depend on the healthy and harmonious functioning of all its limbs and organs. This is also true of the fruitful practice of yoga. When all the components of yoga work together harmoniously, we achieve our goal—attenuation of the afflictions and achievement of samadhi.

In the following sutras, Patanjali describes the specific components of yoga and explains how their mutually supportive functions help us achieve viveka khyati, the highest level of purity and illumination.

SUTRA 2:29

यमनियमासनप्राणायामप्रत्याहारधारणाध्यान-
समाधयोऽष्टावङ्गानि ॥२९॥

yamaniyamāsanaprāṇāyāmapratyāhāradhāraṇā-
dhyānasamādhayo'ṣṭāvaṅgāni ॥ 29 ॥

yama, restraint; *niyama*, observance; *āsana*, physical posture; *prāṇāyāma*, mastery of the pranic force; *pratyāhāra*, recalling the senses; *dhāraṇā*, concentration; *dhyāna*, meditation; *samādhi*, spiritual absorption; *aṣṭau*, eight; *aṅgāni*, limbs

Restraint, observance, physical posture, mastery of the pranic force, recalling the senses, concentration, meditation, and spiritual absorption are the eight components of yoga.

In sutras 1:1 and 1:2, Patanjali and Vyasa tell us that yoga is samadhi, and samadhi is yoga. Samadhi is a state of consciousness in which our core being is fully established in its essential nature. In samadhi we are free of the five afflictions and the pain and sorrow they cause. The techniques leading to this state of realization are also yoga. In "Samadhi Pada," Patanjali introduces several of these techniques but does not elaborate on their specific components. Now he is describing the components of yoga sadhana, and Vyasa is elaborating on their exact functions.

In his commentary on the previous sutra, Vyasa reminds us that the strongest and most deeply rooted among all samskaras is *viparyaya jnana vasana,* our uncompromising loyalty to our mistaken self-identity. This samskara is avidya, the breeding ground for all the other samskaras cluttering our mind. As we practice the eight components of yoga, the impurities originating from avidya, and nurtured by it, are gradually attenuated and eventually destroyed. As both Patanjali and Vyasa explain later in sutras 3:7 and 3:8, the first five components (restraint, observance, physical posture, mastery of the pranic force, and recalling the senses) are the external limbs; and the last three (concentration, meditation, and spiritual absorption) are the internal limbs.

Practicing the external components helps us rid ourselves of impurities that have their source in the external world and have contaminated our body and distorted our behavior. These impurities include those generated by an unhealthy lifestyle, environmental contamination, unnatural breathing, disturbed sleep, and religious and ideological toxins, to name only a few. The internal components—concentration, meditation, and spiritual absorption—help us attain freedom from impurities that have their source in our mental world. Principal among these impurities are our samskaras and the roaming tendencies of our mind engendered and supported by them.

These two categories of impurities always go hand in hand—in the presence of one, the other is bound to form. Similarly, the attenuation of one form of impurity attenuates the other. Mercury poisoning, for example, is an external impurity that causes a variety of physical and neurological disorders which, in turn, are the grounds for mental agitation. To cite another example, sustained fear and anger are internal impurities that destabilize our mind and disrupt many of our physical and cortical functions. The symbiotic relationship between our body and mind causes one form of impurity to give rise to the other. That is why the external limbs of yoga, which have a direct effect on our physical well-being, also greatly enhance our mental well-being. And meditation, which infuses our mind with clarity and stillness, also restores the harmonious functions of our brain and nervous system. For this reason, all eight limbs of yoga are to be applied together—they are listed sequentially only for the sake of study.

In the next twenty-six sutras, Patanjali addresses each of the five external components separately and tells us how to apply them in our daily life.

SUTRA 2:30

अहिंसासत्यास्तेयब्रह्मचर्यापरिग्रहा यमाः ॥३०॥

ahiṁsāsatyāsteyabrahmacaryāparigrahā yamāḥ ॥ 30 ॥

ahiṁsā, non-violence; *satya*, truthfulness; *asteya*, non-stealing; *brahmacarya*, continence; *aparigrahā*, non-possessiveness; *yamāḥ*, restraints

Non-violence, truthfulness, non-stealing, continence, and non-possessiveness are the restraints.

On the surface, it appears that embracing the five restraints—non-violence, truthfulness, non-stealing, continence, and non-possessiveness—helps us build a solid foundation for changing our behavior. They bring out the noble and respectable person in us. We become exemplary and are no longer a source of fear for anyone. These restraints make our life simple, leaving us with plenty of time and energy to attend to our core mission—yoga sadhana. This in itself is a great accomplishment. However, in commenting on this sutra, Vyasa takes the practice of these restraints to a much loftier height.

Vyasa states, "All the restraints and the observances are rooted in *ahimsa*—they are to be practiced to attain perfection in ahimsa." He describes ahimsa as "non-animosity toward all living beings, all the time, and in every respect." This concise statement can be fully understood only in the light of the description of the five afflictions in sutras 2:3–9.

Without exception, all of us are afflicted with fear. All fear culminates in fear of death, which is the epitome of loss. Fear is always accompanied by attachment, aversion, and a false sense of self-identity. It has its roots in avidya and receives its inspiration and nourishment from avidya.

Avidya is our strong attachment to what is contradicted by our intuition. We know the unimaginably vast universe existed long before we were born, and we know the force behind creation is infinitely more primordial, intelligent, and capable than we are. Yet we demand proof. That is the work of avidya. When we are dead, we are nothing. From this nothingness we emerge as a living being. The one who turns the dead into the living and gives us an identity is not only omnipotent but also selfless and infinitely kind. And yet we doubt the incessant flow of its love and guidance. That is the work of avidya. Under the influence of avidya, we defend our self-identity from the primordial omniscient being who breathed life into it in the first place. This avidya-driven urge for self-defense forces us to build a wall around ourselves. This is how *dvaita,* the sense of duality, is born. While living within the confines of duality we are cut off from the immortal, eternal core of our being. The immortal in us is enveloped by the experience of mortality. This is the wellspring of fear. If not checked, it continues perpetuating itself.

Fear is pervasive. We are consumed by the urge to defend ourselves and protect our existence. This urge impels us to take the offensive at the slightest provocation. All living beings—from single-celled organisms to complex entities—are continually emitting their innate fear and filling the objective world with fearful energy. Thus we are living in a world run by fear. The more evolved a creature's intelligence, the more intense and goal-driven is the fear it emits. We humans are highly evolved, so the fear contained in us is more intense and definitive than that in many other creatures. Animals fight and hunt for obvious reasons—procreation and food, for example. We fight for these and for other, subtler reasons—including power, possessions, prestige, and fame. An animal's fear is regulated by nature, so its range of enemies is limited. Our fear is rooted in and propelled by well-crystallized avidya, which has given birth to a highly afflicted mind (Vyasa on YS 2:23). There is no limit to our desires, cravings, ambitions, and urge for self-aggrandizement. This stretches the range of our enemies to an almost limitless size.

Fully formed, fear-driven animosity is a unique characteristic of human beings. It is so subtle and potent that only a person highly endowed with the power of discernment can see its far-reaching, entangled tentacles. Animosity is more subtle than physical or verbal retaliation against a person or a group with the potential to harm us. To describe the subtle nature of fear-born animosity, Vyasa uses a precise term, *abhidroha*, which means "intense aversion that captures our mind from every direction." It is a mental condition that engenders anger toward those we dislike. In other words, intense aversion coupled with anger is abhidroha, the fundamental force behind animosity.

Animosity is always preceded by a strong sense of self-identity. Anyone or anything that threatens our self-identity is our enemy—an individual, an ethnic or religious group, or an ideology contrary to our beliefs. This subtle force of animosity not only makes us shout, shoot our neighbor, and bomb other nations, it also makes us harm our most intimate friend—*buddhi sattva,* the essence of our inner intelligence. That is why Vyasa says that ahimsa is embracing the practice of "non-animosity toward all living beings, all the time, and in every respect."

Vyasa affirms that the remaining four restraints are rooted in ahimsa. When we are not established in ahimsa—in other words, if we have not conquered the primitive urge of self-preservation and thus have not transcended the urge to destroy our "enemy"—we find ourselves under enormous pressure to manipulate our conscience, fabricate evidence, obstruct justice, and do everything possible to justify our intentions and deeds. We are bound to commit *himsa,* violence. This extremely subtle form of himsa is hidden in the deepest recesses of our mind. For untold ages, we have been using this subtle element of violence to defend ourselves and eliminate those who pose a threat to our self-identity. We perceive this as strength. Driven by our subhuman tendencies, we protect and nurture this element at any cost. Misled by this destructive urge, we lie. To hide one lie, we tell ten more. In the process we damage our conscience, hurt others, and disrupt the peace in both our inner and outer worlds.

The same tendency convinces our mind and senses to claim things that are not ours, live recklessly, and consume indiscriminately. This is how we fall from *satya,* truthfulness; engage in *steya,* stealing; get caught up in *abrahmacharya,* sensuality; and become obsessed with *parigraha,* worldly possessions. That is why, according to Vyasa, the remaining four restraints—truthfulness, non-stealing, continence, and non-possessiveness—are rooted in *ahimsa,* non-violence.

As stated earlier, both ahimsa and himsa are extremely subtle. To comprehend the dynamism of ahimsa and himsa, we need a highly refined and perceptive mind. Ordinary people have no capacity even to detect the element of violence at the subtle level expounded by Vyasa. Similarly, embracing the practice of nonviolence at this subtle level is beyond the scope of ordinary seekers. The phenomena of lying, stealing, excessive sense gratification, obsession with worldly possessions, and the ensuing destructive effects on us and on our society are easy to comprehend. By restraining ourselves from lying, stealing, and abusing our senses, and by minimizing our mental and worldly possessions, we are automatically embracing the principle of ahimsa. That is why we practice all five restraints together.

The practice of the five restraints is the foundation for a wholesome life. In spite of the differences in our spiritual, ideological, or professional orientations, we all have a common goal—living a healthy, happy, and fulfilling life. To describe how these restraints serve as the ground for achieving this common goal, Patanjali introduces the next sutra.

SUTRA 2:31

जातिदेशकालसमयानवच्छिन्नाः सार्वभौमा
महाव्रतम् ॥३१॥

jātideśakālasamayānavacchinnāḥ sārvabhaumā
mahāvratam ॥ 31 ॥

jāti, class, *deśa*, place; *kāla*, time; *samaya*, circumstance; *anavacchinnāḥ*, not affected by; *sārvabhaumā*, universal; *mahāvratam*, great vow

[The aforesaid five restraints] are not affected by the factors of class, place, time, and circumstance. They are universally applicable and constitute the great vow.

Yoga sadhana can be divided into two major categories: yoga for aspiring yogis and yoga for those who are accomplished. Aspiring yogis must assess their current physical, emotional, and intellectual capacities before undertaking the practice. They must decide whether mild, intermediate, or intense yogic disciplines are appropriate for them. Accomplished masters, on the other hand, must maintain the highest degree of discipline. In the previous sutra, Patanjali introduces a list of five restraints and Vyasa points out that the first restraint, ahimsa, is the ground for the remaining four, leaving it to us to decide how stringently to embrace them. In this sutra, however, the standard Patanjali sets for practicing the five restraints is applicable to accomplished yogis.

For example, there are two standards for practicing ahimsa.

Killing a human being is murder, but killing a fish is not. Killing a fish is a spiritual offense for a strict vegetarian, but not for a fisherman. Hunting in and around a shrine is an offense, but hunting in the forest is not. For a Hindu, eating meat on the fourteenth day of the moon is an offense, but eating meat on other days is not. In day-to-day life it is a grave offense for a soldier to shoot someone, but it is not an offense for a soldier to kill an enemy on the battlefield.

In the early stages of yoga sadhana, the five restraints—non-violence, truthfulness, non-stealing, continence, and non-possessiveness—can be practiced while paying heed to *jati,* our cultural and professional identities, *desha,* place, *kala,* time, and *samaya,* circumstance, but in higher stages there is no room for compromise. We are expected to embrace these restraints without heeding our class identity, place, time, or circumstance. In higher stages, not only must we practice these restraints in action, we must also practice them in speech and thought. In addition, we must observe the subtle motives behind our thought, speech, and action. This degree of precision and perfection requires supremely refined vigilance. Only *prajna shakti,* the self-revealing power of our inner intelligence, can assess whether or not we have diligently embraced this highly refined practice of self-restraint.

It is important to remember that, in this sutra, Patanjali is describing the characteristics of being established in the unblemished virtues of non-violence, truthfulness, non-stealing, continence, and non-possessiveness. For aspiring yogis, the practice begins with cultivating these virtues until—through consistent practice and self-reflection—we become established in them. Until that time, we practice these restraints as one of the limbs of yoga, continually raising the bar as we become stronger and more enlightened.

In the next sutra, Patanjali introduces the five observances, which constitute the second of yoga's eight limbs.

SUTRA 2:32

शौचसंतोषतपःस्वाध्यायेश्वरप्रणिधानानि
नियमाः ॥३२॥

śaucasantoṣatapaḥsvādhyāyeśvarapraṇidhānāni
niyamāḥ ॥ 32 ॥

śauca, purity; *santoṣa,* contentment; *tapaḥ*, austerity; *svādhyāya*, self-study; *īśvarapraṇidhānāni*, trustful surrender to Ishvara; *niyamāḥ*, observances

Purity, contentment, austerity, self-study, and trustful surrender to Ishvara are the observances.

In the two preceding sutras, Patanjali describes five *yamas,* restraints, which entail actively refraining from violence, lying, stealing, misusing the senses, and hoarding material and emotional possessions. Now he describes five *niyamas,* observances. These entail the active practice of *shaucha,* purity; *santosha,* contentment; *tapas,* austerity; *svadhyaya,* self-study; and *Ishvara pranidhana,* trustful surrender to Ishvara. With these five observances, Patanjali lays the foundation for the remaining six limbs of yoga: asana, pranayama, pratyahara, dharana, dhyana, and samadhi.

Shaucha is of two kinds: external and internal. Maintaining high standards of hygiene, purifying our living space, and keeping our body free of toxins are examples of external purification. Internal purification involves keeping our mind relatively free of karmic impressions and the inner unrest propelled by them.

Not desiring more than we have is santosha. Contentment is both a mental state and a process of being happy with what we have. Without contentment we will never be able to slow the ever-spinning wheel of *karma samskara chakra,* the inexorable process by which mental impressions motivate us to engage in actions that, in turn, further strengthen the mental impressions.

Tapas is withstanding the pain caused by the pressure of the senses and our self-imposed resistance to that pressure. Until we reach the highest, there is a constant tug-of-war between the good and the pleasant, between our discrimination and our desires, between the forces of surrender and the forces of attachment. Cultivating the capacity to withstand this pain and adhering to our resolution is tapas. Observing classic vows, such as *krichchha-santapana* and *chandrayana,* in the way they have been defined by yoga (*yatha-yogam*) is also tapas (Vyasa on 2:32).

Svadhaya involves studying spiritually uplifting scriptures and meditating on a sacred mantra. The study of scriptures connects us with the experiences of previous seekers, and meditation empowers us with direct experience. Together, these two experiences demolish our doubts and free us from fear.

Surrendering our actions and their fruit to the primordial teacher is Ishvara pranidhana. As Vyasa describes it, surrender to Ishvara means maintaining constant awareness of the truth that a higher reality is always with us. It is a reminder that we are not subject to decay and death—experiencing immortality is our birthright. Surrender to Ishvara means seeing that the karmic factors forcing us to remain caught in the cycle of birth and death are dissolving. Ishvara pranidhana is a state of freedom from doubt and fear. Quoting sutra 1:29, Vyasa reminds us that through trustful surrender to Ishvara we succeed in turning our mind inward and attaining freedom from all obstacles.

The five yamas and the five niyamas are subtle. On the surface they seem to constitute a set of yogic ethics. However, a deeper analysis reveals that each of these restraints and observances is an independently powerful practice. Mastering any one of them will accelerate our quest for samadhi, and disregarding any of them will prevent us from moving forward.

How to master these powerful practices and cultivate these great virtues is the subject of the next two sutras.

SUTRA 2:33

वितर्कबाधने प्रतिपक्षभावनम् ॥ ३३ ॥

vitarkabādhane pratipakṣabhāvanam ॥ 33 ॥

vitarka, afflicting thoughts; *bādhane*, arrest; *pratipakṣa*, opposite; *bhāvanam*, thinking

To arrest afflicting thoughts, cultivate thoughts opposed to them.

As long as we have anger and greed, and as long as we are confused about the motivation behind our actions, we will have a negative mind. As long as the five afflictions persist, negative tendencies will flow through our mind. Because most of us have strong samskaras of these afflictions, we know from experience that negative thoughts dominate our mind more easily than positive ones. Our tendency to compete with others, to conquer and attempt to eliminate them, is stronger than our tendency to collaborate with others, to support and embrace them.

As we have seen in sutras 2:4–9, the afflictions are extremely subtle and deeply entrenched. In those six sutras, Patanjali and Vyasa tell us the five afflictions are always present in our mind. Sometimes they are fully active, sometimes moderately active, and sometimes dormant. When they are dormant, we are not aware that the afflictions exist. When they are fully active, they dominate us so completely that our sense of discrimination is swept away. We are aware of being under their influence only when they are moderately active. This awareness provides an opportunity to transform our negative tendencies.

There are numerous negative tendencies powerful enough to agitate our mind and disturb our inner balance. In this sutra, Vyasa uses the example of violence to describe the process of transforming negative tendencies and replacing them with positive ones. Violence is clearly destructive. It springs from fear, one of the fundamental afflictions. According to this sutra, the practice of non-violence requires us to arrest our violent tendencies by cultivating thoughts opposite to violence.

However, if the process of non-violence is to be effective in counteracting violence, we must first describe and outline it clearly and methodically. Because violent thoughts always precede a violent act, an act of non-violence will be effective only if it is preceded by non-violent thoughts. Violence is an active phenomenon, whereas non-violence is mistakenly thought to be passive—simply the absence of violence. But passive non-violence has no power to extinguish the fire of violence. Non-violence must be as active as violence itself.

In an effort to delineate concrete steps for practicing active non-violence, Vyasa describes the process by which violence gathers momentum and finds expression. Before we commit a violent act, a torrent of violent thoughts runs through our mind. For example, the thought arises that a business partner has been diverting money from the firm's accounts. Almost immediately this thought is accompanied by other thoughts: "I trusted this person for years—I thought he was my friend. I have done a great deal for him. I never imagined he would steal from me." This train of thought coalesces in a dichotomy: "I am good; he is bad. I am right; he is wrong." From this arises the desire to punish, laced with the desire for vengeance. We are no longer interested in justice—eliminating the culprit is now our goal. At this point, violence begins to manifest in our speech and action.

In the conventional practice of non-violence we are not led to entertain a stream of structured, organized non-violent thoughts. For example, when someone slaps us on the right cheek, we are told to offer the left one also—this is said to be practicing non-violence. But this approach to non-violence does not free us from pain, nor does it purify our mind. According to Vyasa, we must design a system of practice that neutralizes the force of violence, step-by-step and point-by-point. In violence, the mind is churning out negative thoughts involuntarily. To practice non-violence, we have to train our mind to churn out positive thoughts voluntarily. We accomplish this by the methodical practice of contemplation.

To continue the example cited above, we have to remind ourselves that life is too precious to be consumed by friends and foes, loss and gain. "I have already lost what was lawfully mine. Now I'm allowing myself to lose my inner peace and happiness. This is a much greater loss than losing a portion of my material wealth. Furthermore, such occurrences are commonplace. Everyone has strengths and weaknesses. In worldly matters I will do what needs to be done, but never at the cost of losing the pristine nature of my mind. I must adhere to the higher virtues of my heart." This and similar contemplations cool the heat of violence and help us conserve our mental energy for higher pursuits.

In the next sutra, Patanjali offers guidelines for designing contemplative practices to nullify afflicting thoughts.

SUTRA 2:34

वितर्का हिंसादयः कृतकारितानुमोदिता
लोभक्रोधमोहपूर्वका मृदुमध्याधिमात्रा
दुःखाज्ञानानन्तफला इति प्रतिपक्षभावनम् ॥३४॥

vitarkā hiṁsādayaḥ kṛtakāritānumoditā
lobhakrodhamohapūrvakā mṛdumadhyādhimātrā
duḥkhājñānānantaphalā iti pratipakṣabhāvanam ॥ 34 ॥

vitarkā, afflicting thoughts; *hiṁsādayaḥ*, violence, etc.; *kṛta*, done; *kārita*, made to do; *anumoditā*, consented; *lobha*, greed; *krodha*, anger; *moha*, confusion; *pūrvakā*, preceded by; *mṛdu*, mild; *madhya*, intermediate; *adhimātrā*, exceedingly intense; *duḥkha*, pain; *ajñāna*, ignorance; *ananta*, endless; *phalā*, fruit; *iti*, thus; *pratipakṣa*, opposite; *bhāvanam*, thinking

Violence and the others are afflicting thoughts. We put these thoughts into action by ourselves, through others, or by tacit consent. These thoughts are propelled by greed, anger, or confusion. They are mild, intermediate, or intense. We nullify these afflicting thoughts by realizing they bear unending fruit of pain and ignorance.

In this sutra, Patanjali outlines the dynamics of afflicting thoughts and the destructive actions resulting from them, thus laying the groundwork for a contemplative practice to nullify afflicting thoughts. Using the example of violence, he tells us that these negative tendencies reside in our mind and emerge as feelings. As we entertain them, these feelings gain momentum and demand action. We comply with their demands in three different ways: by involving ourselves directly in an act of violence, by inciting others to violence, or by tacitly consenting to violence. Acts of violence are instigated by greed, anger, confusion, or a combination of these. The consequences of such acts are determined by the intensity of the greed, anger, or confusion that provoked them.

Vyasa outlines eighty-one subcategories of violence according to Patanjali's explanation of the three ways violence is carried out; the three mental conditions of greed, anger, and confusion underlying violence; and the three degrees of intensity—mild, intermediate, and extreme. Vyasa also states that because of the innumerable currents and crosscurrents influencing both our internal and external environment, we express our violent tendencies in myriad ways. The purpose of this elaborate discussion is to help us detect the element of violence in ourselves, identify the instigating factors, and assess their intensity. This will help us design a plan for *pratipaksha bhavana*, cultivating thoughts that oppose and eventually nullify afflicting thoughts.

The cultivation of thoughts contrary to those that need to be eliminated begins with realizing that negative tendencies and actions bear unending fruit of pain and ignorance. Many of us have mastered the art of justifying our negative tendencies and behavior. Once we have mastered the art of ignoring the voice of our heart, we fail to realize that our negative tendencies and behavior have painful consequences. The law of karma, described in sutras 2:12–16, is inexorable. If a negative action is propelled by intense greed, anger, confusion, or a combination of these, and if it is carried out intensely, then—as Vyasa explains in sutra 2:13—unending pain quickly follows. If we somehow manage to escape it in our current lifetime, this pain will manifest as an integral part of our future destiny.

In his commentary on sutra 2:11, Vyasa mentions two kinds of negative tendencies—*svalpa pratipaksha* (little enemy) and *maha pratipaksha* (big enemy). Afflicting thoughts of a gross nature can be easily detected; they belong to the first category and can be destroyed or transformed with the practice of kriya yoga. But afflicting thoughts of a subtle nature, which cannot be so easily detected, belong to the "big" category and can be destroyed or transformed only through meditation.

The desire to eliminate our negative tendencies, both little and big, begins with contemplating the unavoidable consequences of these tendencies. Vyasa outlines one such contemplation:

> Let us see what follows when a killer commits violence. First, he subdues his victim. He damages his victim's self-confidence and self-trust. He puts his victim in a state of fear, thus draining the victim's vitality. Then, he inflicts pain by striking with a weapon. As the pain intensifies, the person dies.
>
> This act of violence has three distinct stages: draining vitality, inflicting pain, and causing death. The karmic consequence will emerge in three distinct stages. The killer must suffer from lack of vitality, strength, and stamina. He must inherit a mind full of fear. He must suffer from low self-esteem. Lacking self-trust, he must rely on the opinions of others and remain indecisive. Because he has inflicted pain, the killer must be born in a species in which, by the design of nature, life is painful. Because he has caused death, the killer must suffer a prolonged and painful death.

This graphic description of a violent act and its consequences should be studied in the light of sutra 2:9, where Vyasa describes the dynamics of death along with the complex process of dying. As we see there, the process of dying brings our conscience forward, forcing us to face ourselves. The moments immediately preceding death present us with an opportunity to see the major theme of our life. We are led to a state of consciousness that affords no room for denying our deeds, what caused us to commit them, and the consequences we will reap as a result. But as we have seen, if practiced correctly, *pratipaksha bhavana* can help us transcend the unending chain of afflictions and reclaim our self-luminous mind.

Vyasa reminds us that the discussion on violence is simply an example—the practice of pratipaksha bhavana applies equally to the remaining restraints and observances. He also reminds us that refraining from bad deeds stops us from creating future bad karmas, but only pratipaksha bhavana—actively practicing the principles which oppose the impressions of afflicting actions—eliminates the root causes of our undesirable destiny.

In the following eleven sutras, Patanjali and Vyasa describe the extraordinary results of practicing pratipaksha bhavana to master the ten restraints and observances.

SUTRA 2:35

अहिंसाप्रतिष्ठायां तत्सन्निधौ वैरत्यागः ॥३५॥

ahiṁsāpratiṣṭhāyāṁ tatsannidhau vairatyāgaḥ ॥ 35 ॥

ahiṁsā, non-violence; *pratiṣṭhāyāṁ*, upon being established; *tat*, that; *sannidhau*, in the presence of; *vaira*, animosity; *tyāgaḥ*, renunciation, absence

In the company of a yogi established in non-violence, animosity vanishes.

In this and the next ten sutras, Patanjali makes a series of bold statements: If you are truly established in the principle of non-violence, the feeling of animosity in those around you will vanish. If you have been practicing truth, your words will materialize. When you embody the principle of non-stealing, prosperity will abide with you. With the perfection of celibacy, you will gain the ability to transmit spiritual power to other seekers. When you adhere firmly to the principle of non-possessiveness, you will gain complete knowledge of the cycle of birth and death. The practice of cleanliness will empower you to detect even the slightest impurity in your body and the bodies of others. That becomes the ground for much higher accomplishments, such as the purification of your core being, cultivation of a positive mind, mental concentration, mastery of the senses, and finally, direct realization. Mastery of contentment will take you to the pinnacle of happiness. The destruction of impurities through austerity will lead you to bodily perfections, such as extraordinary beauty, charm, strength, and self-healing power. Self-study will cause celestial beings to visit you. And, finally, faith in and surrender to Ishvara will grant you the highest yogic reward—samadhi.

It is difficult for those who are not familiar with yoga philosophy and metaphysics to believe that the simple practice of non-violence or contentment, for example, can engender such exalted yogic achievements. Yet these achievements are obtainable because—as Patanjali reminds us throughout the entire text—our core being is absolutely pure and self-luminous. We are different from Ishvara only in the sense that we are caught in the cycle of birth and death. We have been given a wonderful tool—the mind—to discover our relationship with Ishvara and free ourselves from the seemingly unending cycle of transmigration. The luminosity of our mind is identical to the luminosity of our core being. Our mind has inherited all the qualities and powers of prakriti, the intrinsic power of Ishvara.

The problem we face is that at this stage in our evolution our mind and core being have become intermingled. Our mind no longer exhibits the boundless richness of Ishvara and its prakriti. Our mind and core being are enveloped in numberless layers of limitations, such as doubt, fear, and, most important, the subtle impressions of our past experiences. These limitations are outgrowths of avidya, our long-cherished conditioning of self-forgetfulness.

Avidya has veiled our understanding regarding our transmigratory nature, the role of Ishvara in our life, the role of the mind in discovering life's purpose, and the forces that govern and guide our mental and physical activities. In yogic terminology, avidya and its immediate manifestations—distorted sense of self-identity, attachment, aversion, and fear—are known as *kleshas,* afflictions. These afflictions churn our deepest mental tendencies, which, in turn, influence the course of our actions.

Our actions are almost invariably propelled by our deep-rooted afflictions. Subtle impressions created by our actions further reinforce our afflictions. Once fully matured and firmly established, these afflictions dominate the landscape of our consciousness. In response to their demands, we behave compulsively. We act with no understanding of what is happening inside us. This is the point at which the mind becomes decrepit. Its power of discernment dims—it has no capacity to see there is a core being or that its duty is to serve that core being. Not knowing any better, the mind begins to treat this incapacity (*ashakti*) as its prized treasure. This is how the mind loses sight of its inherent *shakti,* the unmatched power inherited from Ishvara's prakriti.

By following the guidelines laid down in sutras 2:33 and 2:34 and by practicing the yamas and the niyamas, we can help our mind free itself from its acquired incapacity and reclaim its inherent capacities. As Vyasa explains in sutras 2:4 and 2:11, the gross forms of afflictions are nullified by practicing *pratipaksha bhavana.* This technique of actively cultivating thoughts opposite to our negative thoughts applies to all the yamas and niyamas. Only an active practice has the power to nullify the gross layers of our afflictions. However, as both Patanjali and Vyasa tell us, the finest and subtlest layers of our afflictions can be destroyed only by meditation.

As the inherent capacities of our mind return, we experience our core being more clearly. We have no doubt about our true identity and are no longer afraid that anything can devour, damage, or even touch our essential self. This level of clarity is enlightenment, the mental state in which the intrinsic luminosity of the mind is no longer obstructed. Armed with its own intrinsic luminosity, the mind begins to command the body, mind, senses, and the entire objective world. Now the practices of non-violence, truthfulness, non-stealing, continence, non-possessiveness, cleanliness, contentment, austerity, self-study, and trustful surrender to Ishvara bear their ultimate fruit.

In this sutra, Patanjali and Vyasa are describing the ultimate fruit of ahimsa, non-violence, the elimination of animosity. Violence is invariably accompanied by fear and anger, which are caused and propelled by desire and aversion. Desire and aversion come from attachment, the mental condition that forces us to cling to our possessions. All of our possessions are contained in the most refined possession of all—our self-identity. Our family, property, religion, intellectual achievement, professional reputation, power, and charisma are all trappings of our self-identity. From the yogic perspective, this is asmita—our distorted sense of self-identity—and it is enveloped in avidya.

For most of us, this distorted self-identity constitutes our personal world. Because this is what we feel ourselves to be, the prospect of losing it is deeply frightening. We do everything in our power to protect and perpetuate our distorted identity. When we fail, we become angry and we direct our anger at people who have harmed us or who have the potential to harm us. This is how animosity is born and how it thrives.

This phenomenon is rampant in both our inner and outer worlds. But at the dawn of enlightenment—another name for the return of our inner luminosity—even the idea of defending and perpetuating our self-identity evaporates. Consequently, attachment, desire, and aversion lose their foundation. As this foundation crumbles, animosity disappears and we are automatically transported to a state of ahimsa.

The maturity of the state of ahimsa depends solely on the practice of pratipaksha bhavana and meditation. How completely the power of ahimsa will nullify animosity in the world around us depends on how elevated our state of ahimsa is and how firmly we are established in it. In addition, the scope and intensity of the collective anger filling the atmosphere have a strong influence on the degree to which non-violence will nullify animosity. In other words, the more pervasive and intense the anger, the larger the group of people established in fully matured non-violence must be. Buddha, Jesus, and Gandhi were all apostles of love and pea ce. All led non-violent movements and all transformed the world around them. Yet they were all killed. This is because the positive energy of non-violence subdues animosity only when it is collectively greater than the negative energy of animosity.

It is important to remind ourselves that perfection in non-violence is an outcome of the highest level of spiritual achievement. It arises as we enter deeper levels of meditation and matures when we taste samadhi. In the context of our day-to-day practice, the principle of non-violence is a powerful tool for transforming ourselves into good human beings and for accelerating our growth, both as individuals and as members of society.

SUTRA 2:36

सत्यप्रतिष्ठायां क्रियाफलाश्रयत्वम् ॥३६॥

satyapratiṣṭhāyāṁ kriyāphalāśrayatvam ॥ 36 ॥

satya, truth; *pratiṣṭhāyāṁ*, upon being established; *kriyāphalāśrayatvam*, the ground for the fructification of the action

When a yogi is established in truthfulness, actions begin to bear fruit.

In this sutra, Patanjali claims that when we are established in *satya*, truth, actions expressed by our words materialize. As with nonviolence, the verity of this claim rests solely on the power of our pristine and self-luminous mind. The mind is innately infused with the powers and attributes of primordial prakriti. Primordial prakriti is infinitely rich in every respect. It is eternally and spontaneously aware of the intention of Ishvara. Prakriti responds to Ishvara's intention, and the world of infinite varieties of matter and energy manifests. In other words, prakriti manifests in perfect accordance with Ishvara. Similarly, our mind responds to the intention of our core being, provided our mind is pristine and pure. Our luminous mind senses our intention instantly. Because the mind has no resistance to that intention, its inherent powers and attributes transform the intention into a living reality.

Words are reflections of our thoughts. Thoughts originate in the depths of our consciousness. Before they turn into action, thoughts flash in our mind as words. When the mind is free from afflicting thoughts and feelings, thoughts and the words corresponding to them flow forth without losing their potency. For example, when Ishvara saw darkness and thought of light, he uttered, "Let there be light," and there was light. When Jesus invoked Moses and Elijah, they appeared instantly.

The science of mantra rests on the principle of revelation, which, in turn, stands on *prajna,* intuitive wisdom. Prajna is not confined by the forces of time, space, and the law of cause and effect; it is beyond the domain of sensory perception, inference, postulation, and even scriptural exhortation. As we have seen in sutras 1:47–50 and 2:27, prajna dawns when the mind is free from afflictions and the mental tendencies arising from them. In this state, truth alone exists.

Riding the waves of the mind's luminosity, truth radiates outward. In this state, only the finest words from the finest of languages present themselves to our mind. Our ultra-refined, enlightened mind selects those words as a conduit to transport the intention of outwardly radiating truth. This is how mantras are revealed. A yogi with direct experience of this process is a *rishi,* a seer. What he experiences is mantra. Because of the pristine nature of the truth, the pristine nature of the intention, the pristine nature of the mind, the pristine nature of the word, and the pristine nature of this entire process, nothing can obstruct, alter, or compromise the transformative effect of mantra. As described in sutra 4:10, the same power is at work in regard to the infallible quality of the blessings of a yogi fully established in truth.

Aspirants who are still attempting to experience this lofty state of truth and become firmly established in it need a methodical practice for applying the principle of truth in daily life. This practice begins with not lying. Once we resolve not to lie, we begin to see the subtle causes of lying. This is when the practice of *pratipaksha bhavana,* cultivating thoughts opposite to those that compel us to lie, becomes applicable. The practice of pratipaksha bhavana in regard to truth begins with reminding ourselves how one lie leads to ten more, embroiling us in an unending cycle of pain and ignorance. Pratipaksha bhavana, coupled with the proper practice of meditation, gradually leads us to a state in which we find ourselves fully established in truth.

SUTRA 2:37

अस्तेयप्रतिष्ठायां सर्वरत्नोपस्थानम् ॥३७॥

asteyapratiṣṭhāyāṁ sarvaratnopasthānam ॥ 37 ॥

asteya, non-stealing; *pratiṣṭhāyāṁ*, upon being established; *sarva*, all; *ratna*, gems; *upasthānam*, coming closer

When a yogi is established in non-stealing, all gems manifest.

When we are established in *asteya,* non-stealing, all gems are drawn to us. Here two terms, *non-stealing* and *all gems,* are extremely significant. *Non-stealing* is more than refraining from the physical act of theft. Non-stealing is a subtle force that seizes our desire to acquire things that are not rightfully ours. This force is infused with discerning wisdom. Just as with practicing ahimsa, practicing asteya requires that we refrain from personally involving ourselves in the act of stealing, refrain from motivating others to steal on our behalf, and refrain from giving our tacit consent.

The second term, *all gems,* denotes more than precious stones. Lofty ideals, scientific discoveries, human values, uplifting thoughts, and the virtues of the heart—love, compassion, selflessness—are invaluable gems. To become established in the principle of non-stealing requires that we refrain from stealing these more subtle gems as well as the obvious ones.

The thought of stealing arises from greed. Greed is an extension of our desires. When desires invade our faculty of discernment—our buddhi—we become consumed by fulfilling them at any cost. Because our buddhi is compromised, we neither see nor care to see the difference between right and wrong. Ethics and morality no longer matter—we are determined to get what we want. To accomplish this, we may involve ourselves directly in achieving what is not ours, employ others to get it for us, or give our tacit consent. To some extent, this has been accepted as a standard business practice. Only when it disrupts the social order are we forced to see what we are doing—pretending that a destructive vice is actually a virtue.

For Patanjali the practice of non-stealing is a requirement of a yogic life. We begin by refraining from taking what is not ours. We refine the practice by not coveting things that are not ours. As our practice becomes even more refined, we become aware of the subtle dimensions of stealing. We realize that a materialistic approach to life, and excessive consumerism, have caused us to plunder resources that belong to future generations.

This realization takes our practice of non-stealing to a new height. Not only are we no longer wasteful, we invest time, energy, and resources in protecting and preserving the future of humankind and the planet. In the subtle realm of divine providence, nature appoints us as custodian of her bounty. As a result, nature's wealth is drawn to us. Celestial bodies shower their blessings on the earth. Rain brings a good harvest; bees produce sweet and nutritious honey; soil exudes fertility; wild fires remain contained; human minds become clear and kind; and we find joy in living in a symbiotic relationship with every aspect of nature. For a self-aware yogi, nature's bounty is a shining gem. When we are established in the principle of non-stealing, these gems are drawn to us and we ourselves are gems.

SUTRA 2:38

ब्रह्मचर्यप्रतिष्ठायां वीर्यलाभः ॥३८॥

brahmacaryapratiṣṭhāyāṁ vīryalābhaḥ ॥ 38 ॥

brahmacarya, continence; *pratiṣṭhāyāṁ*, upon being established; *vīrya*, vigor; *lābhaḥ*, attainment

A yogi established in continence gains *virya*, the capacity to transmit knowledge.

The practice of *brahmacharya* results in the achievement of *virya*, vigor and vitality. Elaborating on this sutra, Vyasa states that the vigor and vitality gained from this practice heal and nurture us to such a degree that nothing can impede the rise of the inherent power and intelligence of our body and mind. We become *siddha*, an accomplished being. As a siddha, we are capable of transmitting knowledge and yogic experience to aspirants who embody humility. In other words, we can guide and awaken our fellow beings through *shaktipata*, transmission of spiritual energy.

Brahmacharya is often translated as "celibacy." It carries a religious connotation and is associated with monasticism. In that context, *brahmacharya* means abstaining from sex in thought, speech, and action. In the yoga tradition, however, the practice of brahmacharya is very precise and methodical. In the Sri Vidya tradition, which is the epitome of hatha yoga, kundalini yoga, and tantra yoga, the integration and nourishment of the three *bindus* form the foundation of brahmacharya. *Bindu* means "dot," and refers to three distinct, yet interconnected, principles that keep us alive and healthy: mind, prana, and virya. As long as these three are fully nourished and working in harmony, our limbs and organs function properly. We have a vibrant and energetic body and are firm and confident.

The practice of brahmacharya enables us to restore the pristine nature of these three bindus and helps us conserve and further enrich their intrinsic powers. In the normal course of life, however, our mental tendencies drain the mind's energy. A shaky, shallow, and noisy breath drains our prana. Sensory indulgence drains our vitality. Mind, prana, and virya are so intricately interwoven that when one is vitiated, the other two are as well. When one is one-pointed, the others become one-pointed. When one is stable and perfected, so are the others.

Yogis of the Natha tradition and those of several other tantric schools employ alchemy to integrate and nourish these three bindus and thereby become established in brahmacharya. The yogis of the Sri Vidya tradition employ the combined methods of hatha yoga, pranayama, alchemy, and mantra sadhana to unite and nurture mind, prana, and virya. The tradition claims that pranayama is the key to the practice of brahmacharya.

Pranayama techniques that help us identify our pranic currents, collect the scattered forces of prana, and allow these forces to travel through *sushumna*, the central channel, to the crown chakra are used for mastering brahmacharya. Most outstanding among all pranayamas in this context are *agni sara, pracchardana vidharana,* and *shambhavi mudra*. These techniques are altogether different from what is taught in standard hatha yoga classes and should be practiced only under the guidance of a competent yogi. When further augmented with the higher practices of mantra, visualization, and alchemy, these pranayama techniques enable us to bring the forces of our mind, prana, and the body's vital energies to a state of balance. We become acutely aware of which particular bindu—mind, prana, or virya—takes the lead in vitiating our focus. With practice, we also learn how to use the other two bindus to control and guide the wayward one.

If need be, experienced masters may confer shaktipata upon us and guide us through the practice until one day we become firmly established in it. At that point, we are able to pass on what we have received from experienced masters—confer shaktipata on prepared students and help them gain a direct experience of what has been lying dormant in their own body and mind.

SUTRA 2:39

अपरिग्रहस्थैर्ये जन्मकथंतासम्बोधः ।।३९।।

aparigrahasthairye janmakathantāsambodhaḥ ॥ 39 ॥

aparigraha, non-possessiveness; *sthairye*, loc. of *sthairya*, firmness; *janma*, birth; *kathantā*, essence of "why"; *sambodhaḥ*, complete understanding

With firmness in non-possessiveness comes complete understanding of the "why-ness" of birth.

Upon gaining firmness in *aparigraha*, non-possessiveness, we unravel the mystery of birth. As we have seen in *The Secret of the Yoga Sutra* (particularly in Appendix C, "The Theory and Practice of Sankhya Yoga") as well as in sutras 2:12–15, our unfulfilled desires bring us back to this world again and again. The desire to be wealthier and more important, and the desire to dominate others and consume more than others, are inherent in all of us. This tendency makes it easier for us to commit violence, be dishonest, steal, and indulge ourselves, rather than to embrace non-violence, truthfulness, non-stealing, and non-indulgence. Behind violence, dishonesty, stealing, and indulgence lies one clear objective—gaining greater control over the objects of our desire and eliminating those with the potential to stand in our way. This phenomenon can be described in one word: possessiveness. We want to have enough to fulfill our desires—and desires know no limit. That is why in the realm of destiny, possessiveness takes a leading role in determining where, how, when, and in what species we will be born.

All of our desires and the possessions corresponding to them belong to one of three categories: *putraishana,* desires associated with family and progeny; *vittaishana,* desires associated with material wealth; and *lokaishana,* desires associated with power and fame. These three categories of desire manifest in numberless ways. When they manifest, they demand action. When we succeed in fulfilling our desires, they demand more. When we fail, we are disappointed, sad, and angry. In both cases, a network of new samskaras is created. Life after life we keep returning to this same cycle.

During the quiet moments of our meditation we can see what type of desire possesses our mind. The object pertaining to that desire is our dearest and most valued possession. If we fail to renounce it, then in all probability that particular possession will take the lead in designing our future life. This process takes place when we are breathing our last. During the time of death, our long-cherished desires and the objects corresponding to them stand before our consciousness en masse. The frail body, depleted brain, and frightened mind are overwhelmed. Finally, the most prominent among all the possessions and desires emerges and dominates our consciousness, and our life force is absorbed into this consciousness. Rebirth is a reversal of this process.

Pratipaksha bhavana, cultivating thoughts opposite to those that most occupy our mind, is the essence of the practice of aparigraha. In practice, non-possessiveness involves renouncing our desires and aversions. Through introspection we come to know what is there to be renounced. With the help of pratipaksha bhavana, vairagya, and meditation, we identify, attenuate, and eventually eliminate our mental possessions, which are forcing us to remain caught in the cycle of transmigration. As we progress in the practice of aparigraha, we begin to see our subtler and more potent mental possessions. We know we must renounce them or they will drag us into yet another helpless birth.

When we are fully established in non-possessiveness, we know that nothing can drag us into the cycle of birth and death. This level of firmness in aparigraha enables us to intuit the mental contents of others. Yogis of this caliber are the perfect guides and torchbearers for seekers. As sutra 1:37 tells us, by focusing on such accomplished yogis we are able to cultivate a peaceful and one-pointed mind.

SUTRA 2:40

शौचात् स्वाङ्गजुगुप्सा परैरसंसर्गः ॥४०॥

śaucāt svāṅgajugupsā parairasaṁsargaḥ ॥ 40 ॥

śaucāt, from purity; *svāṅga*, one's own limbs and organs; *jugupsā*, feeling of impurity; *paraiḥ*, toward others; *asaṁsargaḥ*, unmixing

From purity arises sensitivity to the unclean nature of one's own body; [that leads to] unmixing with others.

SUTRA 2:41

सत्त्वशुद्धिसौमनस्यैकाग्र्येन्द्रियजयात्मदर्शन-
योग्यत्वानि च ॥४१॥

sattvaśuddhisaumanasyaikāgryendriyajayātma-
darśanayogyatvāni ca ॥ 41 ॥

sattva, illuminative property of buddhi; *śuddhi*, purification; *saumanasya*, the essential property of a good mind; *ekāgrya*, one-pointed mind; *indriya-jaya*, victory over the senses; *ātma*, one's self; *darśana*, direct experience; *yogyatvāni*, deservingness; *ca*, and

[From purity arises] the purity of our essential being, a positive mind, one-pointedness, victory over the senses, and the qualification for having direct experience of our self.

Just as he did with the yamas, Patanjali dedicates one sutra to each of the niyamas, with one exception—*shaucha,* purity. His reason for dedicating two sutras to the first niyama becomes clear when we examine them together.

The literal translation of sutra 2:40 is: "From purity [comes] disgust toward one's own body as well as [a desire] not to associate with others." This is confusing because disgust is itself a mental impurity. If that is the result of practicing purity, cultivation of mental purity has no place in the practice of yoga. Only by recalling Vyasa's commentary on sutra 2:32 can we understand how the practice of purity brings forward the feeling of disgust and how that feeling leads to achieving the lofty goals described in sutra 2:41.

The common meaning of *shaucha* is "cleanliness." This covers a vast range of practices running the gamut from daily habits, such as washing our hands, rinsing our mouth, and wearing clean clothes, all the way to extreme practices of fasting, avoiding hearing foul words, and even self-immolation.

Commentators have taken the liberty of selecting a narrow definition of cleanliness and have usually neglected the context in which the concept of purity is introduced in the practice of yoga. Most of these commentators have derived their inspiration from the aspect of Hindu orthodoxy that considers human birth a punishment and the body a vehicle for that punishment. Religious literature that developed in the post-Vedic and Upanishadic period is replete with denigrating descriptions of the body: a lump of filth; a repository of feces, urine, mucus, and bile; a vessel of toxic gas; and so on. In this view, attachment to the body and craving physical pleasure are the grounds for endless misery, while indifference to the body and eventual disassociation from it are the path to salvation. This view is contrary to the very spirit of yoga.

We do not clean our house for the purpose of discovering how dirty it is so we can use this discovery to cultivate disgust for it, and, in turn, use that disgust to motivate us to abandon the house. Similarly, in yoga we do not embrace the principles of cleanliness and purity as a means of cultivating disgust for our body, and then use that disgust to sever our connection with ourselves and with others. Yet only when we begin to clean our house do we notice how pervasive and subtle the dirt is and how deeply ingrained it has become. When we remove the outer layer of dirt, we begin noticing the deeper, subtler layers and can no longer be comfortable living there until we have cleaned the house thoroughly. Similarly, when we begin to follow a regimen for detoxifying the body, we become aware of deeper and subtler levels of toxins and impurities. We become sensitive to the discomfort they cause, and in proportion to that sensitivity we are motivated to stay away from sources of contamination, both internal and external.

In sutra 2:32, Vyasa divides shaucha into two broad categories—*bahya,* external, and *abhyantara,* internal. In general, external purification includes bathing, wearing clean clothes, keeping our home clean and well organized, and infusing our life with sanctity. Internal purity consists of attenuating and eventually eliminating all our mental tendencies, a process that ultimately matures in transcending the five afflictions.

In the yoga tradition, both external and internal purifications are precisely defined and their course of practice clearly delineated. External purification consists of six cleansing techniques known as *shat karma* (see Appendix C). They are *dhauti,* upper wash; *basti,* enema; *neti,* nasal wash; *trataka,* cleansing the cortex with gazing; *nauli,* churning the navel center; and *kapalabhati,* fanning the fire in the head. These six cleansing techniques constitute a significant portion of hatha yoga and are a foundation for the internal cleansing techniques for purifying the mind. In the tantric tradition of Sri Vidya, these external techniques are further augmented with the ayurvedic method of cleansing popularly known as *panchakarma*.

Over the centuries, Sri Vidya masters of the Himalayan tradition continually refined these cleansing techniques. This culminated in a single master practice—*agni sara. Agni sara* means "the essence of fire." With this practice we are able to awaken and capture the internal fire at the *manipura chakra,* the solar plexus (see Appendix D). We also access our pelvic and abdominal cavity and awaken, energize, and nourish our gut brain. The energy generated by agni sara enhances the function of our vagus nerve, which in turn enhances the harmonious function of all our visceral organs. We not only become aware of the toxins and impurities affecting our colon, kidneys, bladder, ovaries, testes, liver, heart, and lungs, but we also cleanse our bodies of those impurities.

Agni sara engenders such a high degree of physical and biochemical cleansing that the harmonious communication and interaction among the central nervous system, the endocrine gland system, the autonomic nervous system, and the internal organs connected to the autonomic nervous system are no longer obstructed by toxins and impurities. Most important, agni sara prepares the ground for practicing pranayama, which opens the door to *abhyantara shaucha,* internal cleansing.

According to chapter 2 of the *Hatha Yoga Pradipika,* our health and longevity depend on the steady, smooth flow of *prana shakti,* the life force. When, with the help of external cleansing techniques, toxins are removed and internal organs energized, the life force flows through the energy channels unobstructed.

The unobstructed flow of prana enables us to clearly observe our deeper states of mind. We know whether or not our mind is disturbed, stupefied, or distracted. We become aware of the factors that rob us of our one-pointedness. We begin to see how fear, doubt, anger, hatred, jealousy, greed, and confusion pollute our mind and motivate us to think, speak, and act irrationally. As Patanjali and Vyasa state in sutra 2:41, this realization motivates us to destroy the deeper causes of these mental pollutants—the five afflictions. As avidya, asmita, raga, dvesha, and abhinivesha are attenuated, we are rewarded with five gifts—the purity of our essential being, a positive mind, one-pointedness, victory over the senses, and the qualification for having direct experience of our true self. We will revisit this subject in our discussion of sutra 2:52.

SUTRA 2:42

संतोषादनुत्तमः सुखलाभः ॥४२॥

santoṣādanuttamaḥ sukhalābhaḥ ॥ 42 ॥

santoṣāt, from contentment; *anuttamaḥ*, unsurpassed; *sukha*, happiness; *lābhaḥ*, attainment

From contentment comes happiness without equal.

Patanjali tells us that *santosha*, contentment, leads to happiness without equal. Elaborating on this sutra, Vyasa says, "All sensual pleasures in the world and the great happiness in heaven combined do not equal even one-sixteenth of the joy that arises from the elimination of craving."

As Vyasa's statement makes clear, practicing contentment means eliminating all craving. Craving is the mature state of desire. There are as many desires as grains of sand on the earth and stars in the sky. These infinite desires are always accompanied by an entourage of fear, doubt, worry, and anxiety. Transcending desires altogether is extremely difficult. As long as we are ignorant of our true identity, and as long as our desires and actions are propelled by deep-rooted mental impressions and tendencies, we are impelled to keep chasing our desires. But there is a way out—contentment.

The practice of contentment begins with a conscious decision not to fixate on the fruit of our actions. It requires a deep conviction that when we perform our actions, the forces governing the law of cause and effect will ensure they bear fruit. When our actions do not appear to bear fruit, we remind ourselves that unknown factors are far more powerful than known factors. When our actions bear desirable fruit, we acknowledge the higher reality that arranges unforeseen factors in our favor. When the fruit is undesirable, we accept it while acknowledging the benevolence of divine will. Thus we remain unperturbed by both the desirable and undesirable consequences of our actions.

In other words, the practice of contentment means recognizing that there is a higher reality, having faith in it, allowing our long-cherished tendencies to run their course, and performing our actions as an instrument of divine will. The more we are established in this practice, the freer we are from the entourage accompanying our desires—fear, doubt, worry, and anxiety. The freer we are from this entourage, the happier we will be.

SUTRA 2:43

कायेन्द्रियसिद्धिरशुद्धिक्षयात् तपसः ॥४३॥

kāyendriyasiddhiraśuddhikṣayāt tapasaḥ ॥ 43 ॥

kāya, body; *indriya*, senses; *siddhiḥ*, yogic accomplishment; *aśuddhi*, impurity; *kṣayāt*, due to the destruction of; *tapasaḥ*, from austerity

Austerity destroys impurities. From that come yogic accomplishments pertaining to the body and senses.

The idea of *tapas*, loosely translated as "austerity," has captured our attention since the beginning of religious history. In every culture, people committed to austerity are perceived as extraordinary and pious. Austerity has invariably been associated with mortifying the flesh for the purpose of subduing or deadening the appetites of the body and senses. This form of austerity includes prolonged fasting, sleep deprivation, self-flagellation, exposure to extreme temperatures, and other forms of self-inflicted pain. In the yoga tradition, practices of this type have nothing to do with austerity and, in fact, are forbidden (*Bhagavad Gita* 17: 5–6).

Commenting on sutra 2:32, Vyasa clarifies that even when they are drawn from the scriptures, practices can be accepted as austerity only when they comply with the fundamental principles of yoga (*yatha-yogam*). *Yoga* means "union." The yogic concept of union applies to every aspect of our being—from the union between mind and body, brain and heart, sympathetic and parasympathetic nervous systems, all the way to the union between Ishvara and the individual self ensnared in the cycle of samsara. Any practice that accelerates the achievement of this union is tapas.

The literal meaning of *tapas* is "shining heat." Tapas is the radiance of the life force—it makes us radiant and vibrant. From the standpoint of practice, gathering and imbibing this radiant force is tapas. To accomplish extraordinary tasks, spiritual luminaries, such as the seven sages, incarnated souls, and celestial beings, like Indra, Shiva, Brahma, and Vishnu, committed themselves to the intense practices of tapas. Only then, as the scriptures tell us, were they able to perform seemingly impossible tasks, such as reclaiming the knowledge unique to extinct races and bringing a century-long drought to an end.

As we saw in sutra 2:18, each of us has the capacity to shine and make the world around us shine. However, most of this capacity has become dormant. Shaking off this dormancy and reclaiming our inherent effulgence is tapas. It has nothing in common with the religious concept of austerity.

In chapter 17 of the *Bhagavad Gita*, Vyasa divides tapas into three broad categories: *shariram*, physical austerity; *vaṅmayam*, austerity of speech; and *manasam*, mental austerity. Observing the principle of purity, practicing humility, observing the principles of continence and non-violence, and committing ourselves to practices that help us reconnect with the pure and transforming power of intuition is physical austerity. Austerity of speech includes speaking only words which are not irritating, are true, are good and useful to others, and, finally, that serve as a means of studying and examining our internal states. Mental austerity is measured by the clarity and joyfulness of our mind. Cultivating thoughts that contribute to the serenity of our mind and fill our heart with kindness fulfill the criteria for mental austerity. It is implemented by observing silence and by observing our thought processes during silence.

As Vyasa states, these three categories of tapas can be sattvic, rajasic, or tamasic. Sattvic tapas, the highest quality, is accompanied by faith. This faith is infused with the highest degree of purity. The practitioner knows the difference between pure faith and blind faith. Furthermore, the sattvic practice of tapas is not tainted by the desire for the fruit of the practice. When we practice tapas with the intention of gaining distinction and attracting attention, it is rajasic. It feeds the ego and its fruit is short-lived. The lowest-grade tapas is austerity carried out by a dull, dense, and stupefied mind. It causes pain and is undertaken out of foolish notions, in defiance of common sense.

This sutra tells us that a high-quality practice of tapas leads to *kaya siddhi* and *indriya siddhi*. *Kaya siddhi* means "bodily accomplishment." According to sutra 3:46, beauty, charm, vitality, and self-healing power are bodily wealth. All of us are born with these four forms of wealth. When both gross and subtle toxins and impurities are removed, our body begins to reveal its inherent beauty, charm, vitality, and healing power. As our practice matures and we become fully established in tapas, a much higher level of bodily wealth—such as the power to become small, big, light, or heavy—manifests spontaneously. The dynamic forces leading to the manifestation of this exalted level of bodily wealth are described in sutras 3:44–46.

The practice of tapas also leads to *indriya siddhi*, perfection of the senses. Our capacity to know the objective world through the senses of hearing, touching, seeing, tasting, and smelling is enormous. But the damaging effect of impurities on our inner intelligence has so eroded the extraordinary powers of our senses that the knowledge we gain through them is limited. The senses regain their extraordinary powers when the impurities blocking the incessant flow of our inner intelligence are destroyed. Our senses then begin to operate in complete conformity with our inner intelligence.

Intuition is another name for inner intelligence. In the realm of intuition, time, space, and the law of cause and effect pose no barrier. Tapas is inner fire. It incinerates the impurities blocking the flow of our intuition. Once these impurities are gone, the power of our senses is unleashed and we begin to comprehend that which lies beyond the domain of our normal perception. In order to understand how this works, let us examine what these impurities are and how they are created.

Impurities fall into two categories: physical and mental. Physical impurities are either toxins created by malfunctioning organs and systems or toxins the body soaks up from outside. Mental impurities are karmic impurities. Patanjali calls them *kleshas*—afflictions—and has elaborated on them in sutras 2:3–11. These deep-rooted impurities churn our mind and manifest as negative *vrittis*—tendencies propelled by anger, hatred, jealousy, greed, and attachment. They pollute the mind, and the polluted mind, in turn, disrupts the natural functions of our body. Both physical and mental impurities disturb the body's natural balance by disproportionately dominating one of the three humors—*vata, pitta,* and *kapha.*

Vata is the fundamental principle of pulsation, movement, and animation. Breath, heartbeat, and cellular respiration are manifestations of vata. Movement, circulation, neurological responses, intellectual processes, expressions of feelings, and creative imagination are a few of vata's many functions. Pitta is the fundamental principle of fire, the force behind transformation. Digestion; assimilation of nutrients; comprehension of information brought to the brain through sensory perception, inference, and postulation, or through revelation; clarity; focus; inspiration; and enthusiasm are a few of the manifestations of pitta. Kapha is the fundamental principle of solidity, the force behind stability and inertia. Kapha reintegrates what has been broken down by pitta.

When they are working in harmony, vata, pitta, and kapha keep us healthy, strong, and energetic. The degree to which their functions are balanced determines the health of our heart, lungs, liver, and other internal organs, as well as the health of our respiratory, circulatory, nervous, and endocrine gland systems.

Vatic disturbances disrupt the normal functions of our heart and lungs, for example, leading to irregularities in heartbeat and blood pressure. From there, a cascade of conditions emerges—congestive heart failure, declining lung capacity, shortness of breath, fluid retention, and a reduced supply of blood to the brain, among others. At the mental level, we become dissipated, erratic, and spacey. Pittic disturbances disrupt our digestive process, overburdening our liver, gall bladder, pancreas, and other organs. Pittic disturbances manifest in acid reflux, ulcers, inflammation of the colon, and skin eruptions. At the mental level, we become irritable, judgmental, fearful, and angry. Kaphic disturbances promote lethargy. We retain fluid and gain weight, and our elimination becomes sluggish. At the mental level, we become dense and dull, our comprehension declines, and we lapse into procrastination and sloth.

In their pristine, balanced state, these three forces sustain our existence. Hence, they are called *dhatu,* the force that holds us together and provides us with nourishment. When imbalanced, they are called *dosha,* defect. A defective body and mind are a burden—we cannot reach samadhi with such a body and mind. Patanjali tells us that cultivating a healthy and energetic body and reclaiming our clear, calm, focused, and intuitive mind is of utmost importance. We achieve this goal by practicing tapas.

Yogis in the Sri Vidya tradition view tapas as *kaya kalpa*. *Kaya kalpa* means "reclaiming the body as it was." It is renewal of the body. Kaya kalpa is a specialty of the yogis belonging to the Sri Vidya tradition. This science derives its inspiration from Ayurveda, Siddha medicine, hatha yoga, and tantra. But the refinement comes from the knowledge of alchemy perfected down through the centuries by the yogis of the Natha tradition. This topic will be elaborated on in the commentaries on sutras 3:38, 3:45–48, 4:1, and 4:4, but a brief discussion of kaya kalpa in the context of tapas will be helpful here.

According to the philosophy and science behind the practice of kaya kalpa, the human body is endowed with extraordinary intelligence and healing power. Its capacity to adapt to the environment and conquer adverse circumstances is matchless. The speed and efficiency with which our endocrine and autonomic nervous systems respond to each other is evidence that our body is designed to defend itself from adverse conditions without burdening our mind with fear and anxiety. Our heart, liver, lungs, kidneys, digestive tract, and brain are centers of intelligence working together to achieve a common goal. This intelligence, which fills every cell and guides and governs the complex system of our body, brain, mind, and heart, is known as *kundalini shakti*.

Kundalini shakti is the primordial pool of power and intelligence. It is the power of all powers, the intrinsic nature of Ishvara. It manifests in us as *prana shakti*. When impurities block the incessant flow of prana, the extraordinary healing and renewing power inherent in our body declines. Communication among the various limbs and organs is disrupted, and the atmosphere inside our body becomes dense and dull. Then the body's systems become confused—they fail to perform their functions effectively, and communication and collaboration among them is disrupted. This unhealthy condition causes our strength, vitality, and stamina to decline. Our love for life erodes—life feels burdensome. Hopelessness sets in, causing the body's innate wisdom to plummet. The immune system becomes weak and dull and the body is susceptible to disease. Kaya kalpa reverses this process and restores the pristine condition of our body and mind.

Kaya kalpa has five main objectives: First, detoxify the five major cleansing organs—colon, kidney, liver, lungs, and skin; second, strengthen the heart and lungs, so they function in a mutually supportive, harmonious manner; third, regulate the digestive system; fourth, energize the solar plexus, to awaken the dormant intelligence of the vagus nerve and to regulate the functions of the visceral and reproductive organs; and fifth, gain access to the space that fills our brain, to energize and strengthen the brain and nervous system.

Tantric alchemy is the core of kaya kalpa. This alchemy is a closely guarded secret. It is far more refined than the herbal formulas of Ayurveda, Siddha medicine, Chinese medicine, and the lost alchemical knowledge of medieval Europe. The tradition prohibits us from exposing the esoteric dimension of kaya kalpa, but permits us to share those portions of this science meant for reclaiming the elements of vibrant health—an elevated level of vitality, virility, stamina, and endurance, and the ability to relax, re-energize, and focus. This dimension of kaya kalpa perfectly blends ayurvedic herbs and nutrition with the asana and breathing techniques developed to accomplish kaya kalpa's five main objectives.

A wise person understands that nothing is more important than reclaiming and retaining vibrant health and so embraces kaya kalpa joyfully. But for a person conditioned by an unhealthy lifestyle, kaya kalpa is a hardship because it requires discipline. Most of us resist change, especially a change in our eating habits. It is equally hard to change habits associated with other sensory pleasures—drugs and alcohol, for example, or entertainment that takes a heavy toll on our body, mind, and senses. But once we get a taste of the vitality of a healthy body and the joy that abounds in a calm and clear mind, we joyfully embrace kaya kalpa as a pleasure and a privilege.

Patanjali and Vyasa tell us this joyful austerity leads to three distinct accomplishments: *kaya siddhi, indriya siddhi,* and *sankalpa siddhi* (YS 4:1). *Kaya siddhi* means "bodily perfection"; *indriya siddhi* means "perfection of the senses"; and *sankalpa siddhi* means "perfection of will and determination."

The human body is naturally endowed with unique qualities and capacities, such as beauty, charm, vitality, and self-healing power (YS 3:46). These qualities are *kaya sampat,* the body's intrinsic wealth (YS 3:45). When the body is freed of impurities and replenished, its innate wisdom awakens spontaneously. Inner balance is restored—our limbs and organs function harmoniously. Our heart, brain, and endocrine and autonomic nervous systems become acutely aware of our internal needs. The healing and nourishing process is accelerated. The internal organs are revitalized. The sense organs and the subtle power and intelligence that empower them with the capacity to comprehend, feel, and act are energized and responsive. This is *kaya siddhi,* the perfection of the body.

Kaya siddhi is the beginning of *indriya siddhi,* perfection of the senses. When the body is free of impurities, the power and intelligence of the senses flow freely through the sense organs. Although the sense organs are the instruments of seeing, tasting, touching, hearing, and smelling, the actual power to see, taste, touch, hear, and smell is contained in our brain, the physical manifestation of our mind. The power that enables the eyes to see, the tongue to taste, the skin to transmit the sensation of touch, the ears to hear, and the nostrils to smell is prana shakti. Once the impurities are removed, prana shakti flows throughout the body unobstructed, empowering our senses to function at the speed of our mind (YS 3:48). Our senses are able to comprehend our thoughts, feelings, concerns, decisions, and, most important, our intentions, and are able to translate them into action instantly. This ability is indriya siddhi.

Bodily perfection and perfection of the senses prepare the foundation for *sankalpa siddhi,* perfection of will and determination. Once we have regained the original purity of our body and senses and they are fully replenished, they begin to function at full capacity. Every cell, tissue, and organ in our body is lit by the inner luminosity of our mind. Our sense organs and the deeper intelligence that infuses them with special powers and privileges conform to the feelings and intentions of our mind. Our habits and cravings lose their grip on our senses, so our sensory activities and biological urges do not contaminate the decisions and resolutions made by our higher intelligence.

Furthermore, because our body and senses are purified, healed, and revitalized, our memory becomes sharp and stable—what we have decided to accomplish remains firmly in the forefront of our consciousness. Now that we know the capacity of our body, mind, and senses has no limit, we are confident we will be successful in anything we decide to do. Self-confidence and self-trust free us from fear and doubt, so we are able to invest ourselves fully in achieving our goals. This is sankalpa siddhi.

To ensure that the extraordinary accomplishments manifesting from tapas are used wisely for the furtherance of our inner growth, Patanjali next introduces svadhyaya.

SUTRA 2:44

स्वाध्यायादिष्टदेवतासम्प्रयोगः ॥४४॥

svādhyāyādiṣṭadevatāsamprayogaḥ ॥ 44 ॥

svādhyāyāt, from self-study; *iṣṭa,* desirable, capable of guiding and enlightening; *devatā,* intrinsic power of *deva,* the bright being; *samprayogaḥ,* union with

From self-study comes the opportunity to be in the company of bright beings [of our choice].

In sutra 2:1, Patanjali selects the last three niyamas—tapas, svadhyaya, and Ishvara pranidhana—from the vast body of yoga and collectively assigns them an independent term, *kriya yoga.* This is clear evidence that these three niyamas play a key role in enabling us to succeed in our practice. In the same sutra, Vyasa emphasizes tapas, telling us, "For those not committed to tapas, yoga does not bear fruit." He does not emphasize svadhyaya, but simply describes what Patanjali means: "Japa of mantras with purifying capacity, such as the mantra *om,* and the study of scriptures is svadhyaya." But here Vyasa addresses self-study in detail.

This sutra reads, "Self-study gives us the opportunity to be in the company of bright beings of our choice." Vyasa adds, "Bright beings are the *rishis* and the *siddhas.* They visit those committed to svadhyaya and take part in their work." Most commentators did not elaborate on this sutra, and the few who did simply repeated Vyasa's statement. Scholars have taken pains to decipher which particular god Patanjali has in mind and, therefore, which god is most likely to visit the practitioner committed to self-study. These discussions and the underlying premise are contrary to the fundamental concept of Ishvara.

In sutras 1:24–29, Patanjali posits the concept of Ishvara. Patanjali's Ishvara is radically different from the idea of God conceived by the various religions. Ishvara is not an individuated entity. It is all-pervading, omniscient being. It is beyond time, space, and the law of cause and effect. It does not fit into any category. Ishvara is an absolute reality. It is beyond cognition—the mind and senses cannot comprehend it. This reality does not visit anyone, for it permeates all times, places, and entities. We may or may not see it, but Ishvara is always seeing us. For this reason, Patanjali and Vyasa avoid using *Ishvara* in this sutra and instead use *ishta devata,* which can be loosely translated as "deity of our preference." Therefore, the most precise translation of this sutra is, "Self-study results in having *darshana* of the deity of our preference." The literal translation of *darshana* is "seeing, comprehending." Thus, according to Patanjali, self-study gives us the capacity to see and comprehend the deity of our choice.

It is important to note that this deity is not Ishvara exactly, for it carries a hint of individuatedness and Ishvara does not. As we will see in the following discussion, this ishta devata—a deity who, due to self-study, walks into our life—does two things: it pulls Ishvara toward us, and it pushes us toward Ishvara. This is when the highest samadhi dawns.

Let us see how the yoga tradition views the idea of deity and how self-study gives us the ability to see and be in the company of the deity of our choice. The term for deity used in this sutra is *devata*, and it is further qualified by the term *ishta*. *Devata* means "essence of deva, essential attribute of deva." *Deva* means "shining being, bright being." Thus *devata* means "the essential attribute that makes a bright being bright." In other words, the intrinsic brilliance of shining beings is devata. The word *ishta* means "that which is chosen." Thus *ishta devata* means "the essential brilliance of the bright beings we choose to imbibe."

This sutra tells us that self-study empowers us to be in the company of devas, beings characterized by their inherent unalloyed luminosity. In yoga, theses devas are the masters belonging to the category of *videha* and *prakritilaya* (YS 1:19, 1:48–50, 2:18, 3:54–55, and 4:29–34). During their lifetime, these masters are established in *dharma megha samadhi.* After death, they become an integral part of Ishvara's intrinsic prakriti. At the behest of divine will, these accomplished beings emerge from prakriti. Because they are free of the five afflictions, their knowledge—the power of knowing—is absolutely pure and unobstructed. They have the ability to see both the unmanifest and manifest spheres of reality. Because they are transcendent beings, time and space pose no barrier to their comprehension. This is why these self-luminous immortal beings are called *rishis,* seers.

Like the rishis, mantras are immortal beings. The only difference is that the body of rishis is made of pure light while the body of mantras is made of pure sound. In the tantric tradition, this is called *nada,* more precisely *anahata nada,* unstruck sound. Unlike sound in the empirical world, anahata nada is not dependent on physical matter or energy as its source or conduit. Like rishis, mantras emerge at the behest of divine will. In their purest form, they are not perceptible to our senses and ordinary mind. Someone who is as pure as the mantras can intuit them. Such pure beings are videha and prakritilaya yogis. Because these beings see the mantras as they are, they are called *rishis,* seers.

It is important to understand exactly what these seers see—the radiance of self-luminous beings, who, at the behest of Ishvara, use the purest form of unstruck sound as their locus. After being seen by the seer, this radiance is known by the name imparted by the seer. For the sake of communicating with others, that seer conceives a form with identifiable attributes. This is how a devata is "born." This devata, in essence, is pure radiance, yet it has a name and a corresponding form.

As we saw in sutra 2:1, engaging in mantra japa and contemplating on the contents of scriptures dealing with subjects such as mantra, seer, devata, and our relationship with them is svadhyaya. When we do japa of a particular mantra for a long time, without interruption, and with reverence, we eventually reach a high level of mental absorption in the mantra. The technical term for this is *mantra samapatti.* In this state, the radiance of the mantra, along with the name and form conceived by the seer, begins to dawn on the horizon of our awareness. Furthermore, the essence of the seer—the power of seeing itself—occupies our awareness along with the seer's name and form. This is what this sutra means by stating that svadhyaya results in a vision of the deity of our choice. Elaborating on this sutra, Vyasa states that bright beings, sages, and accomplished masters visit the practitioner of svadhyaya and take part in his work.

In other words, mantra japa gives us the ability to see the shakti inherent in the mantra. As mantra japa ripens, the rishi and devata belonging to that mantra rise on the horizon of our consciousness. Although we are in their full view and they in ours, our long-cherished samskaras, preferences, and mental conditioning cloud our vision. Yet just as we know the sun is shining even on a cloudy day, we feel the presence of these radiant beings—mantra devata and rishis—even when filtered through the clouds of our samskaras. However, we do not comprehend them exactly as they are. Our cultural, religious, and samskaric conditioning dim and often distort the purity of the experience. We comprehend the name and form of the radiant shakti in direct proportion to the quality and capacity of our mind. This is why the same divinity is seen as very beautiful, less beautiful, terrifying, fully human, or partially human, with one face, three faces, two arms, or even eight or ten arms.

In the beginning stages, experiences pertaining to the rishi and devata may be fleeting and occur only in dreams. These experiences may be so mingled with our mental tendencies we may not see any spiritual value in them. Due to the dense darkness of tamas during sleep, we may not even remember these experiences on awakening. And yet if we sincerely and consistently engage ourselves in the practice of the yamas and niyamas—most importantly tapas—we purify and expand the quality and capacity of our mind and eventually receive a clearer, purer vision of the seer and the devata of the mantra. This vision will be free of anthropomorphic projections because it will not be obstructed by our mental conditionings. Even in our waking state we will be able to experience the subtle counterpart of the divine radiance—*nada*, unstruck sound, and *bindu*, self-luminous light.

Each time we gain these experiences, our capacity expands, until one day we are able to comprehend the essence of the divinity and the sage who embodies it. At this stage, our connection with the seer and the radiant being the seer sees is fully and firmly established.

Those who have reached this level of realization are called *siddhas,* the accomplished ones. The radiance illuminating them becomes the locus for their consciousness when they are in meditation, and that same radiance is available to them after they cast off their body. They continue living as luminous beings but are not absorbed in the intrinsic prakriti of Ishvara like the rishis, and therefore are not as omniscient and pervasive. But neither are they buried in the dense darkness of death. They are fully awake, and the matter and energy that constitute the empirical world pose no barrier. As sutra 3:32 tells us, the radiance of siddhas is not confined to the earthly plane.

Self-study enables us to see and live in the company of bright beings—rishis and siddhas—who are inherently imbued with brilliance. Here "brilliance" refers to the transforming power of their intrinsic luminosity. In the presence of this radiance, we not only see these luminous beings but we also begin to sense and eventually experience our own inherent radiance. Each time we come in touch with these bright beings, our consciousness is elevated to a new height. Their presence fills our consciousness with ever-greater purity, thus destroying the veil that hides our *buddhi sattva,* the essence of our inner intelligence. We comprehend reality as it is.

At the unveiling of our buddhi sattva, we are able to comprehend Ishvara and Ishvara's intrinsic prakriti. Our fear of dissolving into Ishvara's prakriti vanishes. We no longer see Ishvara outside us or ourselves outside Ishvara. We realize the guiding grace of Ishvara has always been with us, and that this divine grace grants us lasting fulfillment and ultimate freedom. With humility and gratitude, we spontaneously surrender to Ishvara. This opens the floodgate of the highest samadhi, the subject addressed in the next sutra.

SUTRA 2:45

समाधिसिद्धिरीश्वरप्रणिधानात् ॥४५॥

samādhisiddhirīśvarapraṇidhānāt ॥ 45 ॥

samādhi, state of mind beyond all cognition; *siddhiḥ*, yogic accomplishment; *īśvara*, all-pervading divine being beyond time and space and absolutely untouched by affliction; *praṇidhānāt*, from trustful surrender

From trustful surrender to Ishvara comes samadhi.

Before we examine the idea of trustful surrender set forth in this sutra, it is important to remember that Patanjali dedicates seven sutras to this subject in "Samadhi Pada" (YS 1:23–29). Here he is repeating sutra 1:23 almost verbatim. This is significant because the tradition of sutra-style writing demands that the author avoid repetition and be absolutely succinct and precise. So let us see what Patanjali, one of the most notable pillars of the tradition, is communicating with this repetition.

Here Patanjali is quite precise in regarding trustful surrender as the doorway to the highest samadhi. Back in "Samadhi Pada," immediately after introducing the idea of trustful surrender to Ishvara, Patanjali enters into a prolonged explanation of the nature of Ishvara (YS 1:24–26). Only then does he state that Ishvara is represented by mantra and explain how mantra japa turns our consciousness inward and removes obstacles (YS 1:27–29). As these seven sutras make clear, Ishvara is absolute being—beyond time, space, and the law of cause and effect. It has no form and no name and it is omniscient. In the world comprehensible to our senses and mind, there is nothing parallel to Ishvara's distinctiveness. Thus it is indescribable. How can we surrender ourselves to something we do not and cannot know? Only when we read sutra 2:45 as a continuation of sutra 2:44 and augment it with the experiences of the yogis who have traveled this path do the concepts of trustful surrender to Ishvara and divine grace opening the door to samadhi become comprehensible.

For all intents and purposes, *rishis*, the seers, are Ishvara. The ordinary mind can only go this far. But as we continue our mantra sadhana, our mind becomes increasingly infused with the seeing power of the seer. Our ordinary mind is transformed into *buddhi sattva,* the extraordinary mind, for we have regained our unalloyed luminous intelligence. With this fully transformed mind we are able to see the seer in her fullness. We are able to see the seer's oneness with Ishvara, for we too have become seers.

Our mind is no longer "our" mind—it is the mind of the seer. Now we see the totality of the truth through the eyes of the seer. This "seeing" is utterly different from any form of seeing and knowing familiar to us in the objective world. The understanding that dawns in this state is as unique as the seers themselves. The experience is all consuming. It annihilates all mental tendencies and deep-rooted afflictions—ignorance, distorted self-identity, attachment, aversion, and fear. All curiosity regarding who we are, where we came from, where we will go after we die, and how long we will stay in the company of the sage that blessed us with this unique experience vanishes. As we saw in sutra 1:51, this is how we reach the highest samadhi gracefully and spontaneously.

In the Sri Vidya tradition, the highest-caliber seer is called *maha preta. Maha* means "great"; *preta* means "gone forever" and refers to one who is dead. *Maha preta* is one so well dead there is no possibility of being reborn. Brahma, Vishnu, Shiva, Rudra, and Ishana are maha pretas. They are depicted as the "couch" of the nameless, formless, indescribable, transcendent being. In his concluding sutra (YS 4:34), Patanjali calls this transcendent being *chiti shakti,* the power of consciousness.

In the Sri Vidya tradition, chiti shakti is known as the divine mother, Sri Vidya. These five maha pretas—the highest-caliber seers—are absolutely absorbed in her. There is no difference between chiti shakti and these enlightened beings—they are one and the same. From the standpoint of our practice and experience, they are the locus for the all-pervading absolute. They are so intrinsically one with the absolute that the notion of them as one or many has no meaning. They are timeless and thus as unborn as the transcendental Ishvara, yet their appearance marks the beginning of time. That is why such a seer (*rishi*) or cluster of seers (*rishi gana*) is called *sadyojata*, born instantly. The seeing power is also known as *vama deva*, the bright being who makes the unmanifest manifest.

It is the seeing power of these divine beings that sees the mantras. In essence it is the seeing power of pure consciousness and as such there is only one seer, Ishvara. Figuratively speaking, rishis are the eyes of Ishvara. The attempt we make to see Ishvara through the eyes of these rishis is yoga sadhana. When we invest all our physical and mental resources in our practice—most importantly in the practice of tapas and svadhyaya—and become exhausted by our self-effort, we are automatically in a state of surrender.

According to the *Bhakti Sutra* of Narada, the state of surrender is not engendered by our self-effort (BS 1:7). Surrender is not dependent on our desire or plan—it dawns on its own. The only thing that precedes the experience of surrender is *mahat kripa,* the grace of the great souls—the seers (BS 3:38). The seers do not plan to confer their grace on us. Grace is absolutely unconditional. It is *durlabha,* hard to acquire, but once acquired its effect is *amogha,* unfailing. We receive and retain grace only through grace. Upon receiving it, we see grace everywhere—the gift of life is grace, living in the world is grace, and attaining freedom from the cycle of birth and death is grace. We are thrilled that we ourselves have become the eyes of the seers, and we know beyond doubt that the seers and what they see are one (BS 2:39–41 and 4:55). This realization frees us from all desires, including the desire to attain samadhi. That is when the door to samadhi opens.

It is important to remember that this extraordinary achievement, *samadhi siddhi,* is the result of an extraordinary level of trustful surrender. This is an experiential state, one we reach only when we commit ourselves to a methodical practice. Each of us has our own starting point. Where we start our practice of trustful surrender depends on how clearly we comprehend svadhyaya and how sincerely, fearlessly, and joyfully we embrace the guiding grace of the divine being. We comprehend the transforming power of this guiding grace in proportion to the purity and discerning power of our mind, which largely depends on the practice of tapas. Thus these three—tapas, svadhyaya, and Ishvara pranidhana—go hand in hand and together breathe life into all the other limbs of yoga. Without these three, the yamas and niyamas remain confined to the realm of ethics and morality. Asana remains a set of exercises for enhancing physical health. Pranayama will improve our vitality, strength, and stamina, nothing more. Pratyahara is merely an excellent tool for relaxing our nervous system. And although dharana, dhyana, and samadhi will enhance our mental concentration, they will have little or no spiritual value. In the light of this understanding, Patanjali next explores the remaining eight limbs of yoga.

SUTRA 2:46

स्थिरसुखम् आसनम् ॥४६॥

sthirasukham āsanam ॥ 46 ॥

sthira, stable; *sukham*, comfortable; *āsanam*, posture

A stable and comfortable posture is *asana*.

At first glance, this sutra does not seem particularly significant—simply by being steady and comfortable we accomplish the third limb of yoga. This appears to indicate that there is a disconnect between the rigors of the yamas and niyamas—especially tapas, svadhyaya, and Ishvara pranidhana—and asana, which is characterized by steadiness and comfort. We are steady when resting on the couch and comfortable when asleep in bed. Is Patanjali including asana in the system of yoga as casually as it sounds in this sutra? What about Vyasa, who confines his comments to listing a few sitting postures by name without bothering to explain what asana actually is? What are we missing?

As he did in sutra 1:36 of "Samadhi Pada," here Patanjali compacts a thousand years of collective experience into a single sutra. Over millennia, the yogis have developed hundreds of techniques to master their body and mind, and used that mastery to accomplish life's purpose. Some of these techniques remained narrow in scope, while others expanded to such an extent that they came to be treated as an independent discipline. That is how various schools—such as kundalini yoga, tantra yoga, laya yoga, mantra yoga, bhakti yoga, karma yoga, jnana yoga, and hatha yoga evolved. They all adopted the fundamental techniques of hatha yoga. In fact, it is the inclusion of hatha yoga techniques that defines the physical, mental, and spiritual disciplines of all these schools as yoga. Patanjali's system of yoga is no exception.

Asana lies at the heart of hatha yoga. The simplest meaning of *asana* is "posture." Within the context of hatha yoga, posture means arranging our limbs and organs so our body becomes acutely aware of the forces of *ha* and *tha*. In yogic literature, *ha* and *tha* stand for solar and lunar, or masculine and feminine energy, respectively. When combined with other techniques of hatha yoga—such as pranayama, bandha, mudra, and dharana—the practice of postures increases our sensitivity to solar and lunar energies while unblocking, balancing, and further nourishing these energies. There are hundreds of postures in the hatha yoga tradition.

When Patanjali adopts the asana component of hatha yoga as an integral part of his *ashtanga yoga*—the eight-limbed yoga—he is assuming his readers have a fundamental knowledge of hatha yoga and are fairly well established in its practice. Vyasa lists only sitting postures, because here asana is introduced in the context of yoga as a means for reaching samadhi, which requires sitting in meditation for a prolonged period.

The most popular term for the eight-limbed yoga set forth by Patanjali is *raja yoga*, "the royal path of yoga." *Raja* means "royal, stately." Its lofty status is due to its balanced and highly evolved inclusiveness. All meaningful philosophies and practices belonging to other schools of yoga are included in one or another of the limbs of raja yoga; the entire range of hatha yoga practices are subsumed in three of these limbs: asana, pranayama, and pratyahara.

According to tradition, when asana, pranayama, and pratyahara are practiced in the light of the yamas and niyamas, hatha yoga emerges as a fully developed spiritual path. The transformative power of hatha yoga engenders a positive change in our worldview as well as in our body and mind. When the techniques for meditating on the chakras are added, hatha yoga assumes a new identity—kundalini yoga. But when hatha yoga embraces the techniques of dharana, dhyana, and samadhi, it emerges as raja yoga. In other words, raja yoga is the full expression of hatha yoga—and much more. Thus, in the *Hatha Yoga Pradipika,* Svatmarama proclaims, "It is not possible to master hatha yoga without raja yoga or raja yoga without hatha yoga. Therefore, one should practice them together." (HYP 2:76).

In this and the next two sutras, Patanjali describes the dynamics of asana, which builds the foundation for the practices of pranayama and pratyahara. In conjunction with pranayama and pratyahara, the practice of asana prepares the ground for the practices of dharana, dhyana, and samadhi, the last three limbs of ashtanga yoga.

The practice of asana described in this sutra is grounded in the philosophy outlined in sutra 2:18. According to that sutra, the objective world is composed of elements and the senses that enable us to perceive them. The objective world is imbued with the powers of illumination, action, and stability and has a twofold purpose—fulfillment and freedom. The objective world made of matter and energy is unimaginably vast. In contrast, our personal world is made of our body and mind, which are relatively small and easily accessible. For all intents and purposes we are our body and mind. Nothing in the universe is nearer and dearer to us. All the great powers and privileges described in sutra 2:18 are buried in our body and mind. By discovering that wealth and investing it wisely, we accomplish life's purpose—lasting fulfillment and ultimate freedom. The science of discovering and reinvesting the inherent wealth of the mind is described in the third chapter of the *Yoga Sutra,* "Vibhuti Pada." But how to discover and reinvest the intrinsic wealth of our body is the subject of this chapter.

The discovery of the infinite wealth buried in the body begins with asana. The technical term for this wealth is *kaya sampat.* Patanjali describes the vast range of kaya sampat in four major categories: *rupa,* beauty; *lavanya,* charm; *bala,* vigor and vitality; and *vajra-samhananatva,* inner healing power (YS 3:45–48).

The first category of bodily wealth is *rupa,* beauty. All of us have an innate sense of beauty and so we are naturally drawn to beauty. Our urge to be beautiful has no limit. The evolution of our physical form stretches far beyond the Darwinian demands for survival and procreation. At different stages of life our body expresses its innate beauty in different ways. In response to this expression we make various gestures, assume different postures, and adorn ourselves with various garments and ornaments. Landscaping, architecture, interior design, and the fine arts are all extensions of our inherent beauty. This intrinsic passion for beauty and the desire to be acknowledged as beautiful set us apart from the rest of creation.

The second category of bodily wealth is *lavanya,* literally "the essence of salt." Lavanya refers to the quality of tastefulness. It is a quality that brings out our inner charm, which has an insatiable urge for continued refinement. It motivates us to envision and create an environment that offers more than what we need to sustain our day-to-day existence. This is the quality that enables us to form and maintain a family, society, culture, religion, and other socio-political groups. Because of this quality, our scope of betterment is continually expanding.

The third category of bodily wealth is *bala,* vigor and vitality. Like beauty and charm, our vigor and vitality is limitless. Our body is smaller than that of many other creatures but the strength, stamina, endurance, patience, enthusiasm, and courage we embody are far more expansive. Our vigor and vitality are highly refined and full of intelligence. This intelligent, vital force has an irresistible will to express its limitless capacities. For example, it gives us the vision and the courage to move faster than any other creature, and to fly higher. Compelled by this force we invent machines and transfer our vigor and vitality into them. Just as our hands, feet, and sense organs are an extension of our inner intelligence and operate in response to it, so are our machines. There is no limit to the expressions and functions of this vital force.

The last category of bodily wealth is *vajra-samhananatva,* inner healing power. All of us are imbued with vajra-samhananatva, adamantine indestructibility. Like vigor and vitality, this healing power is extremely refined and intelligent. It is *amrita,* the elixir of immortality. The antidote to decay and death, it keeps disease and old age at bay. Our finite body is the container of this infinitely vast healing power. It pervades every nook and cranny and supports all our physical and biological activities. The functions of our internal organs all the way to our mitochondrial and biomolecular functions are expressions of this inherent healing power. Like our vigor and vitality, this healing power has the irresistible urge to express itself in a limitless manner. In response to its calling, we continuously discover and refine healing modalities. Herbal formulas, antibiotics, nuclear medicine, and spiritual healing techniques, such as mantras and rituals, are a few examples of the invincible character of our inner healing power. It sustains our love for life and fills us with trust that one day we will defeat disease, old age, and death.

Even though we are born with an infinite wealth of beauty, charm, vigor, vitality, and healing power, we suffer from self-denigration, loneliness, physical and mental depletion, and fear of disease, old, age, and death. According to Patanjali, all this suffering is avoidable provided we discover the cause and delete it. We are living in a body imbued with vast potential, and yet our mental faculty is so dull and dense that we are only dimly aware of its internal dynamics.

We have become disconnected from our body's intrinsic intelligence. This dims our recognition of our inherent beauty, charm, vigor and vitality, and healing power, and eventually blocks their flow completely. As a result, our ability to be happy with what we are and what we have, our ability to embrace all and exclude none, our ability to cultivate and retain a robust and energetic body, and our ability to heal ourselves and each other plummet. This disconnection also disrupts the incessant flow of information among the body's various systems and organs, and so they begin to function chaotically. This is how we become unhealthy and succumb to disease. A diseased body demands constant attention—we busy ourselves caring for it and have no time or energy to enjoy living in it. But as soon as we restore our connection with our body, our inner balance and harmony return. We become healthier, and we have ample time and energy to discover the purpose of having a human birth.

Restoring the natural connection with our body and reestablishing inner balance and harmony begin with the practice of asana. Stability and comfort are the hallmarks of yoga postures. Stability arises when a limb, organ, or system is not disturbed by the functions of other limbs, organs, or systems. In an overtly frightening situation, for example, our sympathetic nervous system triggers a rush of adrenalin. The heart beats faster to meet the demand for increased blood supply in the area actively engaged in countering the threat. If this situation continues for an extended period, we hyperventilate: the heartbeat accelerates, the nervous system becomes shaky, and the endocrine system is thrown out of balance.

Fear is pervasive. No human is absolutely free of fear. As long as it does not manifest with overwhelming force, we may pretend it does not exist. That is why there is always some degree of instability and shakiness in our body, breath, senses, and mind. As soon as we restore our inner balance and harmony, a large range of physical conditions no longer pose an obstacle to our spiritual quest.

Similarly, comfort comes when a particular limb, organ, or system is not stressed by the functions of other limbs, organs, and systems. For example, when lung capacity declines, the volume of oxygenated blood flowing from the lungs to the heart also declines. The heart must pump harder and faster to meet the demand of the body and brain. This stresses the heart, causing general discomfort in the body. A pose that removes this stress and enables us to experience the pleasure of having a comfortable body is considered to be a yoga posture.

Over millennia, yogis invented thousands of postures—some highly significant and others less so. Eighty-four are considered classic. Commenting on this sutra, Vyasa enumerates only thirteen postures, and all of them are sitting postures. This is because the goal of raja yoga is samadhi. Samadhi begins with meditation, which can be practiced only in a sitting posture.

However, it is important to remember that the qualities of stability and comfort, which make a sitting posture a yoga posture, are cultivated by the practice of asana as taught in the tradition of hatha yoga. In order to cultivate a steady and comfortable sitting posture, we must take our body through a range of postures—including standing, bending, sitting, reclining, twisting, and inversions. Only then does the practice of asana energize and restore the harmonious functions of all our limbs and organs. And further, we must practice asana methodically, in the proper sequence, and after meeting all the prerequisites.

In the following sutra, Patanjali delineates the golden rules for refining and perfecting both sitting and non-sitting postures.

SUTRA 2:47

प्रयत्नशैथिल्यानन्तसमापत्तिभ्याम् ।।४७।।

prayatnaśaithilyānantasamāpattibhyām ॥ 47 ॥

prayatna, special effort; *śaithilya,* a stress-free state; *ananta*, infinite; *samāpatti*, mental absorption

[Perfection in asana is attained] by loosening of [tension caused by] effort and by [mental] absorption in the infinite.

In this sutra, Patanjali lays out the criteria for perfection in asana. According to him, precision is more important than how long and how vigorously we practice. Precision in asana practice has two components. First, the effort involved must not cause fatigue or create tension. Second, when we reach the peak of the posture we must stay there for a while and allow our mind to be absorbed in the space that fills our body and the space surrounding us.

Practicing asana effortlessly is a subtle and highly technical process involving motion. The law of inertia states that an object at rest tends to stay at rest and an object in motion tends to stay in motion, unless a contrary force is exerted on that object. An object resists the exertion caused by a contrary force. During the practice of asana, we need to apply the force of will to pull our body out of its initial inertia. Following the law of physics, the body will pass through the moment of inertia, which is the time required to overcome its initial inertia and move. In relation to an inert object, the moment of inertia is quantifiable and the subsequent change is easily predictable. The moment of inertia can be also quantified in relation to our body, but because it is imbued with will and intelligence, the subsequent motion is not easily predictable. The subtle forces of will and intelligence grant us the privilege of increasing or decreasing the resistance to motion; therefore, we can choose to practice asana with significant effort or with relatively less effort.

Effort causes resistance, resistance engenders tension, and tension constricts our cells and tissues. Constricted blood vessels cannot supply sufficient nutrients to our limbs and organs, nor can constricted cells absorb sufficient nutrients from the blood. Furthermore, constriction stiffens our connective tissue, causing a reduction in the overall elasticity of our body. If we apply force, it will cause pain; pain further intensifies tension. If we persist in applying extra effort, we may injure ourselves. The lesson we learn from that is not to make an effort while practicing asana. But if we do not make an effort, how can we advance in our practice? The solution is to make an effort effortlessly. Here is how.

First, find the baseline of your comfort. To do this, lie on your back, relax, and breathe gently and smoothly. As you pay attention to the gentle, even flow of your breath, your heart, lungs, and other internal organs relax. Your nervous system and brain calm down, and your connective tissues soften and become smooth. After a few minutes, gently get up and do some simple stretching. This will bring your body to a place where you will be able to assess your baseline comfort.

Now move into your desired posture. For example, if you are practicing the standing forward bend, bend forward until you approach your threshold of discomfort. Do not go beyond your current range of flexibility and strength but stay just at the threshold of your discomfort. In other words, continue bending forward until you reach the point where your brain is just beginning to register a physical and mental response. If you have not reached the threshold of discomfort, your brain will not register a response.

Stay in the pose effortlessly, which is possible only when you are breathing diaphragmatically without holding tension in the lower back, pelvis, or abdominal area. Each time you inhale—and especially when you exhale—you will notice that you are bending further effortlessly. If you are not making a deliberate effort to move deeper into the stretch and if your attention is on the smooth, gentle, even flow of your breath, you will know when you are just about to cross the threshold of your discomfort. That is the time to start slowly moving out of the pose. Returning to an erect posture will require some effort, but you can minimize it by coordinating your movement with your inhalation. This is what Patanjali means by *prayatna shaithilya*, effortless effort.

Each time we repeat this practice, we cross our previous threshold of discomfort comfortably. In other words, practicing a posture effortlessly pushes the threshold of discomfort further away, allowing the range of our comfort to expand. In this expanded comfort zone, we are able to experience the stability of our posture.

Stability and comfort go hand in hand, allowing us to remain relaxed during the peak moments of the posture. Because we are relaxed, the tissues in the area directly engaged by the posture are not constricted but are free to receive and assimilate the nutrients delivered by the increased blood flow. This accelerates the healing process. We become stronger and more flexible and energetic. Our stamina and endurance expand. Due to the lack of pain, our mind is free to concentrate on the space that occupies the region of the body most directly affected by the pose, in this case the lower back and the pelvic and abdominal cavities. This is when the second principle leading to perfection in posture, *ananta samapatti*, mental absorption in the space, applies.

The literal meaning of *ananta* is "without an end." The most common meaning is "space." In yoga, tantra, and Indian mythology, *ananta* refers to the *shesha*, primordial serpent, the absolute remainder. Ananta is the all-pervading intelligence of pure consciousness. It is self-existent and does not require anything as its locus. Rather, its pervasiveness is the locus for everything that exists. In the human body, this all-pervading, self-existent intelligence is indicated by the term *kundalini shakti*. It is the substratum of what we are, the source of all forms of healing power, and the ground for longevity. Just as mitochondria run and regulate our metabolism, kundalini shakti supports and guides the general functions and activities that sustain life. Kundalini shakti is the subtlest of all forms of energy. It has no corollary in the world of matter. It is *chidakasha*, pure space, intelligence without form. It fills every nook and cranny of our body.

When we are able to stay in a posture effortlessly, we employ our mind to enter the space in the area most directly affected by the pose. This, too, is to be done effortlessly. Through prolonged, uninterrupted practice we reach a point of complete mental absorption in that space. Following the principle laid down in sutra 1:41, this absorption infuses the mind with the intelligence of that space. Thereafter, the cascade of transformation begins. The mind becomes as bright and intelligent as the space occupying that area of the body. It becomes acutely aware of the strengths and weaknesses in that area. This awareness further energizes that region and guides the mind in seeing how to overcome those weaknesses. In response to this mental awareness, the brain—in conjunction with the autonomic nervous system and the endocrine gland system—accelerates the process of cleansing and rejuvenation. The end result is that we become clearer, stronger, and more intuitive.

When we practice a broad range of asana precisely for a long time while observing all the prerequisites, we acquire sufficient strength and stamina to endure and eventually transcend all physical and emotional pain. That is the subject of the next sutra.

SUTRA 2:48

ततो द्वन्द्वानभिघातः ॥४८॥

tato dvandvānabhighātaḥ ॥ 48 ॥

tataḥ, from that; *dvandva*, pair of opposites; *anabhighātaḥ*, lack of injury

From that [comes] lack of injury caused by the pairs of opposites.

Patanjali proclaims that mastery over asana enables us to remain free from injury. This is a monumental claim. Vyasa makes an even bigger claim: After attaining victory over asana, a yogi is no longer subdued by the pairs of opposites, such as heat and cold and the many other pleasant and unpleasant experiences that walk into our lives.

The claims made by these two masters are grounded in a long of tradition of yogis who risked their lives for the furtherance of yoga, particularly the practice of asana and pranayama. The practices that many of these yogis committed themselves to were so extreme and intense that modern-day practitioners might consider these adepts to be yoga maniacs. For example, some tested the perfection of their asana by practicing *trataka*—focusing their gaze directly on the sun. Others practiced *pancha agni* by focusing their mind at the navel center while surrounded by fire in all four directions, with the midday sun blazing overhead. Some practiced *kumbhaka*, breath retention, for hours or days while focused on one of the major chakras.

These practices led them to develop sharp and far-reaching vision, the ability to remain unaffected by extreme heat and cold, and the capacity to live a long time free of disease. But collectively, they paid a high price—many lost their lives while experimenting with these and other extreme practices. However, such experiments and experiences led them to conclude, "A yogi grounded in asana takes a dip in the fountain of bliss comfortably and happily" (*Shiva Sutra* 3:16).

According to Vyasa and Patanjali, bathing in the perennial fountain of bliss is preceded by a yogi's ability to transcend pain. Asana enables us to transcend pain only when we practice it in accordance with the rules laid down in the previous two sutras.

There are thousands of postures. In order to heal our physical and psychological injuries we must learn to select the postures suitable to our specific needs and arrange them in the proper sequence. Sequencing of asana is crucial because, as with anything else, a change in sequence drastically changes the result (YS 3:15). Next, we have to practice these properly sequenced postures while staying within the boundaries of our comfort. Then, we must take our practice to the point where we are able to feel and touch the threshold of our discomfort. We refine our practice as we apply the principle of effortless effort described in the previous sutra. This refinement enables us to cross the threshold of discomfort comfortably. In this way, the range of our comfort continues to expand until we are prepared to practice asana with a high degree of intensity.

Due to the application of effortlessness, our body is fluid and we are able to move in and out of a posture easily and comfortably. This in itself is a major accomplishment. But bringing the claims of Patanjali and Vyasa within the realm of our personal experience requires that we enhance the intensity of the practice. To do this, we must voluntarily apply resistance.

We take a big leap when we augment the intensity of our practice with the power of resistance. In this light, yogis in the Sri Vidya and Natha traditions have selected a series of asanas that are simple enough for anyone, but when the intensity is increased and resistance is applied, these simple postures influence our body and mind at a totally different level. Intensity and resistance are applied by combining asana with the practices of pranayama, bandha, and mudra. This high-intensity sequence of asana, further augmented by a high degree of resistance, culminates in one master practice—*agni sara.*

As we see in Appendix D, agni sara subsumes all the elements of asana, pranayama, bandha, and mudra. It leads our body through what is known in today's fitness world as high-intensity interval training, and it does so while staying within the yogic parameters of stability and comfort. Furthermore, agni sara forces us to apply a high degree of resistance while adhering to the principle of effortlessness. In the advanced stages, it also gives us an opportunity to direct our awareness to the region of the body most affected by the contraction and expansion engendered by the alternating forces of resistance and relaxation.

Agni sara has a direct effect on the major organs involved in cleansing and detoxification—the colon, kidney, liver, and lungs. The practice demands that we pull our perineum; skeletal muscles; connective tissue; ligaments; the tendons directly or indirectly connected to the coccyx, sacrum, hip joints, and pelvis; and the abdominal cavity in and up as we exhale, and allow them to relax and return to their normal position as we inhale. This forces our diaphragm to move vigorously. The enhanced performance of the diaphragm and lungs strengthens and regulates the functions of our heart. Lifting the energy from the lower chakras, concentrating it at the navel center, and further churning it under the enormous compression created by agni sara awakens our inner fire, boosts our autonomic nervous system (particularly the vagus nerve), and regulates and nurtures our visceral organs. The force with which we push our spinal fluid upward toward our brain and then allow it to flow effortlessly downward is not found in any other yoga practice. It is no wonder that for centuries yogis have been using agni sara as a means to reverse aging.

Put simply, this master practice fills our body with vitality, strength, and stamina. Agni sara energizes all our internal organs. It enhances and balances the functions of the central and autonomic nervous systems. It restores the link between our heart and brain. It awakens cellular intelligence, particularly in the region of our abdomen and intestines. Agni sara makes us robust and energetic, thus allowing us to reclaim our extraordinary immune system. Pleasant and unpleasant experiences—both physical and psychological—can no longer disrupt the ecology of our body and mind. We become stable and comfortable in our body—a quality we must cultivate in order to practice pranayama. That is the subject of the next sutra.

SUTRA 2:49

तस्मिन्सति श्वासप्रश्वासयोर्गतिविच्छेदः
प्राणायामः ॥४९॥

tasminsati śvāsapraśvāsayorgativicchedaḥ prāṇāyāmaḥ
॥ 49 ॥

tasmin, after that, upon that; *sati*, only then, never without; *śvāsa*, inhalation; *praśvāsayoḥ*, dual possessive of *praśvāsa*, exhalation; *gati*, movement, speed; *vicchedaḥ*, cessation, elimination, stopping, controlling; *prāṇāyāmaḥ*, composite of *prāna* and *āyāma*, expansion of the life force

Complete mastery over the roaming tendencies of inhalation and exhalation is *pranayama*; it is to be practiced only after mastering asana.

This is one of those sutras where the nature of language prevents us from deciphering the precise meaning without help from a living tradition. According to the rules of Sanskrit grammar, *pranayama* means "expansion or stretching of *prana,* the life force." The process of expanding our life force, according to this sutra, is accomplished by *gati-viccheda,* stopping the movement of our inhalation and exhalation. By following another equally valid grammatical formula, the expansion of the life force could also be accomplished by disconnecting the movement of inhalation from the movement of exhalation. Both interpretations are counterintuitive. After all, when inhalation and exhalation stop, we die. When the movement of inhalation is disconnected from the movement of exhalation for a prolonged period, we die. Death and expansion of the life force are mutually exclusive. What are we missing here?

The first two words of this sutra, *tasmin* and *sati,* solve the riddle. Together, they mean "only then." "Only then" refers to the content of the three preceding sutras, which are dedicated to the practice of asana. In other words, the dynamics of pranayama described in this sutra and the practice of pranayama elaborated on in the upcoming sutras can be comprehended only after we have mastered asana.

Perfection in yoga comes from attaining mastery over the mind and prana. Mind and prana are twin and mutually dependent laws—they go together. When one is disturbed so is the other. The stability of one stabilizes the other. Mastery over the mind does not mean arresting our mind, nor does mastery over prana mean arresting our prana. In sutra 1:2, Patanjali says that we attain mastery over the mind by arresting its roaming tendencies. Here he tells us we attain mastery over prana by arresting its chaotic functions.

Prana is the fundamental principle of pulsation. It is the primordial ripple of the life force—beginningless and unending. It is self-intelligent. Like primordial prakriti, prana is both unmanifest and manifest. In its unmanifest state, it is referred to as *kundalini shakti*. Prana manifests in response to Ishvara's will—it is the vibrant, intelligent force that breathes life into matter. Prana is not our creation—we are its creation. It is as pervasive as Ishvara and as omniscient. Following divine will, prana manifests in us in different grades and degrees. As humans we have been given the power and privilege to further awaken and gather *prana shakti* and thus fill ourselves with a higher degree of vigor, vitality, strength, stamina, and intelligence. We accomplish this through the practice of pranayama.

Pranic pulsation fills every nook and cranny of our body. The functions of our cardiac muscles, lungs, and diaphragm are its expressions. The movement in our limbs and organs and the functions of our senses are reflections of pranic pulsation. However, the most tangible and identifiable movement of prana is the breath. From the physical and biological standpoint, *prana* means "breath." Every aspect of our body is directly connected to the breath. We are able to sustain our body and bodily functions only as long as we breathe. Even a minor fluctuation in our breathing pattern disrupts the body's normal functions. According to *yoga shastra,* by regulating our breath we regulate all our biophysical processes.

Working with the breath is subtler than working with the body, which is why pranayama requires a higher degree of training than asana. By the same token, pranayama is far more rewarding. However, pranayama can be practiced only after we are established in asana. It is also important to remember that the scope of asana is limited if it is not accompanied by pranayama. In tandem, asana and pranayama mature into the higher stages of yoga, which culminate in samadhi.

The practice of pranayama begins with arresting our irregular breathing patterns. The breath is the link between the body and the mind, as well as the balancing factor. When a disturbing thought arises in the mind, our breathing pattern becomes erratic—shaky, noisy, and shallow. Erratic breathing triggers a chaotic response in our nervous system, gastrointestinal tract, endocrine glands, and heart. If left unchecked, the chaotic response intensifies, throwing us into a state of physical and mental turmoil. This process can be checked only if the breath summons its innate wisdom and the power to calm itself. Calming the breath involves breathing deeply and evenly, without jerks or noise. Deep, even breathing restores the body's natural equilibrium. However, if the breath fails to summon its innate wisdom and power, we breathe mechanically. The heart and brain will still attempt to meet the demands of our limbs, organs, and systems, but because mechanical breathing is bereft of inner intelligence, the healing and nourishing functions of breathing will be highly compromised. According to this sutra, arresting the mechanical movement of the breath and infusing the breath with conscious awareness is pranayama.

The heart of pranayama practice is *prana samrodha,* methodical restraint of prana. This is the process by which we identify, capture, and pull pranic movement to a designated area of our body and confine it there. Because prana is so subtle as to be imperceptible to an untrained mind, we begin by developing sensitivity to our breath in a particular region of our body, such as the navel center, heart center, or the region between the tip of the nostrils and the eyebrows. The yogic term for cultivating sensitivity to the subtle counterpart of physical breathing is *prana samvedana.*

The practice of prana samvedana entails learning to feel the breath's natural movement and experiencing how the breath is affecting a particular region. Prana samvedana enables us to identify and pinpoint the details of subtle breathing, which in the normal course of life remain imperceptible to our mind. The process of identifying and pinpointing these subtle details is technically known as *prana anusandhana.* The practice of prana anusandhana consists of a set of seven pranayamas: *aharana pranayama, samikarana pranayama, dirgha-prashvasa pranayama, nadi shodhana pranayama; anuloma pranayama, viloma pranayama,* and *pratiloma pranayama* (see Appendix E.)

These seven pranayamas are not designed to arrest the movement of our breath and confine it to a particular region. Instead, they help us become friends with our breath, strengthen our breathing apparatus, identify the baseline of our comfort in breathing, approach the threshold of our discomfort, and at some point—just as in the practice of asana—enable us to cross the threshold of discomfort comfortably. These seven pranayamas help us cultivate the vigor, vitality, stamina, and endurance we need for the more advanced pranayama practices, all of which include breath retention. These advanced practices are the subject of the following sutras.

SUTRA 2:50

बाह्याभ्यन्तरस्तम्भवृत्तिर्देशकालसंख्याभिः
परिदृष्टो दीर्घसूक्ष्मः ॥५०॥

bāhyābhyantarastambhavṛttirdeśakālasaṁkhyābhiḥ
paridṛṣṭo dīrghasūkṣmaḥ ॥ 50 ॥

bāhya, external; *ābhyantara*, internal; *stambha*, stopping wherever it is, immobilizing; *vṛttiḥ*, movement; *deśa*, space; *kāla*, time; *saṁkhyābhiḥ*, numbers; *paridṛṣṭaḥ*, fully seen, properly monitored; *dīrgha*, long; *sūkṣmaḥ*, subtle

[Pranayama with breath retention could be] threefold: external, internal, or stopping the breath wherever it is. Each is monitored by space, time, and number, and each is characterized by its length and subtlety.

Patanjali describes three kinds of pranayama: *bahya,* external; *abhyantara,* internal; and *stambha,* stopping wherever it is. Each involves *kumbhaka,* breath retention. Holding the breath after completing an exhalation is external kumbhaka; holding it after an inhalation is internal kumbhaka; and holding it suddenly in the midst of either an inhalation or an exhalation is *stambha vritti kumbhaka.*

These three advanced pranayamas are steps toward meditation and samadhi. Patanjali assumes that aspirants who have reached this level of yoga sadhana are familiar with the practice of the seven pranayamas, which together constitute the practice of *prana anusandhana* (see Appendix E). Therefore, these aspirants have built a strong foundation for practicing the three advanced pranayama techniques he is presenting here. Let us see how to practice them.

We will begin with external breath retention. Establish yourself in a comfortable sitting posture. Exhale gently and slowly, without noise or jerks. When your exhalation is complete, close the nostrils with your fingers and hold your breath to your full capacity; then release the nostrils and inhale gently, slowly, smoothly, and soundlessly. At the end of the inhalation, exhale slowly and repeat the cycle. This process must be monitored by space, time, and number.

Monitoring by space means becoming aware of the region of the body where you feel your exhalation begin. As you continue exhaling, your breath moves away from the place where it began until it reaches a particular point in the space outside your body. Maintain awareness of that point in space while retaining your breath. At the culmination of the retention, begin inhaling from the exact point in space where you confined your breath outside your body, and continue until you reach the space inside your body where your exhalation began. At the completion of your inhalation, begin the next cycle of external retention. This is how external breath retention is monitored by space.

Practicing external breath retention while observing the area covered by the practice, both inside and outside your body, is easy for those who have practiced the seven prana anusandhana practices, but difficult for those who have not. If you have not mastered these seven pranayamas, you will merely be imagining the space. Traveling through this imaginary space will compromise the efficacy of the practice or nullify it completely.

Monitoring by time means timing the movement of your exhalation, retention, and inhalation. In other words, in addition to maintaining awareness of where in the body your exhalation began, how much space it covered before it reached its destination point outside your body, and then how your inhalation returned to the point of origin, you also pay attention to the time involved.

As a general rule, you retain your breath twice as long as you exhale, and inhale for one quarter as long as you retain—a ratio of 2:4:1. For example, if it takes 20 seconds to exhale, retain the breath for 40 seconds, and while inhaling, cover the same space in 10 seconds. This is to be done without noise, jerks, or discomfort.

Monitoring by number is the next step. Even though Patanjali mentions number as a tool for monitoring the breath, in practice, counting is used to measure the time of the inhalation and exhalation. To preserve the 2:4:1 ratio, you could count from 1 to 20 while exhaling, from 1 to 40 while retaining, and from 1 to 10 while inhaling. However, using numbers will cause two problems. First, the words representing numbers are not of equal length. For example, it takes longer to pronounce "seven" than it does to pronounce "one," and pronouncing "twenty-seven" takes even longer. So using numbers to measure the time covered by the exhalation, retention, and inhalation will disrupt the 2:4:1 ratio. In subtle practices like these, failing to preserve the ratio can be detrimental to your health and mental clarity. The second problem with using numbers to monitor time is that no matter how silently you count, the mental articulation of the words corresponding to the numbers will create jerks in your breath, compromising its smooth, even quality and distracting your mind from its total engagement with space and time.

The solution? Coordinate the exhalation, retention, and inhalation with your mantra. Every mantra has a specific number of syllables. Because Sanskrit is phonetic, each syllable requires the same length of time to pronounce. Therefore, if you remember your mantra four times while exhaling, eight times while retaining the breath, and twice while inhaling, you will preserve the 2:4:1 ratio. However, you must be so well practiced with your mantra that the sound flashes in your mind effortlessly and thus causes no fluctuation in your breathing.

The second pranayama described in this sutra is internal kumbhaka. This is similar to the external kumbhaka described above, except here you inhale first, retain, and then exhale, while following all the rules laid out for external kumbhaka.

The third pranayama, stambha vritti kumbhaka, is the most complex and difficult. In this practice, you retain your breath in the midst of the inhalation or the exhalation. Retaining your breath in the midst of an inhalation is easier than retaining it in the midst of an exhalation. Retaining the breath in the midst of both inhalation and exhalation is extraordinarily difficult, but mastery of it—as yogis proclaim—enables an adept to conquer death.

Let us see how to do the simplest version of stambha vritti kumbhaka. Make sure that you adhere strictly to the standard rules for monitoring your inhalation, retention, and exhalation by space and time. As always, inhale gently and smoothly, without noise or jerks. In the midst of inhaling, stop your breath and retain it four times longer than you inhaled. Then inhale again, filling your lungs fully, and retain again, four times longer than the second inhalation. At the end of the second retention, exhale twice as long as both inhalations combined. As you can see, monitoring your breath by the number of mantras is crucial in the practice of stambha vritti kumbhaka. This entire process must be accomplished without exertion. Take a few normal breaths, then repeat the cycle again.

Practicing these three kumbhaka pranayamas expands the field of inhalation, exhalation, and retention. We are able to inhale, exhale, and retain our breath for a longer period of time (*dirgha*) without discomfort. Furthermore, as the practice becomes refined (*sukshma*), we are able to feel and touch our *pranamaya kosha,* the pranic sheath that supports our body internally. We become aware of the deeper dimensions of our existence. Using the power of prana shakti, which rules our inner world, we are able to take our mental clarity and concentration to a new height.

The three pranayamas described in this sutra constitute a complete practice leading to the awakening of kundalini shakti and are the exclusive domain of kundalini yoga. When kundalini shakti awakens, our limited pool of prana shakti expands spontaneously. It renders even the deepest karmic impressions inert. Our karmic impurities are burned, the energy channels are purified, and the mind enters *sushumna,* ever-pulsating divine luminosity. We are submerged in the primordial pool of kundalini shakti. This is what the practitioners of kundalini yoga consider samadhi. It is an extremely demanding path.

As a student of raja yoga, our goal is to cultivate a clear, calm, tranquil, and one-pointed mind. We then turn this calm and one-pointed mind inward and allow it to bathe in the luminosity of our core being. The longer our mind is infused with the luminosity of our core being, the less chance we have of being affected by our deep-rooted habits. We recapture our innate power of discernment and gain the strength to face and conquer our most dreaded samskara—avidya. To help us accomplish this, Patanjali prescribes a simple, yet highly potent, pranayama in the next sutra.

SUTRA 2:51

बाह्याभ्यन्तरविषयाक्षेपी चतुर्थः ॥५१॥

bāhyābhyantaraviṣayākṣepī caturthaḥ ॥ 51 ॥

bāhya, external; *ābhyantara*, internal; *viṣaya*, domain; *ākṣepī*, that which transcends; *caturthaḥ*, fourth

The fourth pranayama transcends the domain of external and internal pranayamas.

The pranayama described here is far more potent for a meditator than the three pranayama practices described in the previous sutra, because it evolves directly into pratyahara, dharana, dhyana, and samadhi. This pranayama is simple—anyone can do it. However, those who are convinced that an advanced practice must be complex and strenuous will fail to grasp the advanced and highly refined quality of this pranayama.

Patanjali and Vyasa do not give this pranayama a name but simply call it *chaturtha,* which means "the fourth." In the philosophical literature of India, "the fourth" is highly significant. Other terms for *chaturtha* are *turiya* and *turya*. In philosophical literature, *chaturtha* has been used to denote the reality or state that transcends the triangle of waking, dreaming, and dreamless sleep; Brahma, Vishnu, and Shiva; Kali, Lakshmi, and Sarasvati; the powers of will, knowledge, and action; earth, heaven, and the space in between; the three states of the power of speech: *pashyanti, madhyama,* and *vaikhari*; and the three universal processes of creation, maintenance, and destruction. In short, *chaturtha* means "transcendental, the highest." By calling this technique *chaturtha pranayama,* Patanjali is sending a clear message: its effect transcends the vigor, vitality, and transforming power engendered by the three pranayamas discussed in the preceding sutra.

As we will see in the following pages, success in chaturtha pranayama depends on our ability to become aware of our breath and the subtle force of prana that propels it. Those with a body free of toxins and a mind free of roaming tendencies will find it easy to become aware of the flow of prana shakti in their body. But most of us commit ourselves to yoga sadhana only after we have disrupted the natural ecology of our body and thrown our mind into turmoil. A sluggish body and a dense mind are not fit to practice yoga. And yet this is where most of us begin. Thus even though chaturtha pranayama is not dependent on what we gain from the three pranayamas described in the previous sutra, they have an important role to play in preparing many of us for practicing it.

The human body can be compared to an ocean. The ocean is saturated with life-supporting nutrients, most of which are available only where the water is not stagnant. Thousands of undercurrents churn the nutrients and carry them from one part of the ocean to another. Our body and mind are like that. Nature has deposited enormous sustenance—prana shakti—in us. It is available to every cell, because numberless undercurrents—*nadis*—churn our prana shakti and carry it to all our tissues. When this process slows, our limbs, organs, and mind suffer from diminished prana, and the vitality of our body and the sharpness of our mind decline. Many of us, especially those beset by sloth, inertia, fear, uncertainty, confusion, and purposelessness, are so cut off from the flow of prana that our senses and mind have lost much of their acuity. Feeling the flow of prana shakti as part of the practice of chaturtha pranayama is therefore out of reach. In these cases, the pranic force inherent in the body has to be churned and the nadis have to carry it throughout the body so that the senses and mind regain their natural acuity.

When we commit ourselves to a disciplined practice of one or more of the three pranayamas discussed in sutra 2:50, prana shakti begins to churn throughout the body. This churning is most palpable in the region stretching from the perineum to the center of the forehead.

The inhalation and exhalation portions of these pranayamas energize and unblock the energy channels and pull prana shakti out of its inertia. Upon awakening, prana shakti rises upward. The retention portion of these pranayamas gathers the fire of prana shakti and fills the region of the body directly interacting with the retention. As we repeat the practice, the fire of prana shakti intensifies in the region of the body where the breath is being retained. As soon as we resume normal breathing, the process of equalization begins. This is a natural physiological response—the concentrated prana shakti in the region where the breath was retained rushes into parts of the body where it is less concentrated. If we are vigilant, we will feel the movement of prana shakti along the prominent pathways of the energy channels. Because the prana shakti is concentrated, it flows with greater intensity, strength, and velocity, pushing aside impurities.

When we repeat the practice after an interval of a minute or two, prana shakti is churned, awakened, and flows toward the region of the body where we intend to retain the breath. This time, the prana shakti moving toward the region of breath retention is much freer and more forceful, so the concentration of prana in the region where the breath is retained is greater than before. At the end of the cycle, the prana shakti will flow into the rest of the body with even greater strength and velocity. In this way, these advanced pranayamas churn our physiology and biochemistry, burn impurities, and supply nutrients to every limb and organ. But these are only the physical benefits.

According to the yogis, the true benefit of these advanced pranayamas is that they engender a highly captivating energy field, which pulls the mind toward it like a magnet. Upon entering this highly charged pranic field, the mind begins to take on the intrinsic qualities of prana shakti. Prana shakti is the life force—the intrinsic power of Ishvara. In its unmanifest form, it is kundalini shakti. Intelligent and self-luminous, it is the source of all healing power. It is the inexhaustible elixir of life. The *Yoga Vasishtha* calls it *brahma-spanda,* pulsation of the absolute (YV 25:3). When united with prana, our mind begins to move in conformity with the pulsation of the prana. This enables us to become aware of the space our body occupies and of the limbs and organs comprising our body. We become acutely aware of the deeper dimensions of ourselves. The mind and body are no longer strangers to each other (YV 11:52).

The churning and concentration of prana shakti is best accomplished with the practice of *pracchardana vidharana pranayama* described in the commentary on sutra 1:34 in *The Secret of the Yoga Sutra: Samadhi Pada.* As we saw there, because pracchardana vidharana is one of the most advanced pranayamas, it involves a number of prerequisites and preparatory practices. Students of meditation will get the same or similar results by practicing chaturtha pranayama, provided they make an ardent effort to grasp its subtlety and simplicity. In regard to chaturtha pranayama, how long we practice makes very little difference—what matters is how precisely we practice. Here is a brief description of how to do chaturtha pranayama.

Assume a sitting posture suitable for you. Withdraw your mind from every direction and become aware of your body and the space it occupies. Make sure your spine is straight, your shoulders are relaxed, and there is no arch in your lower back. In an attempt to keep your head, neck, and trunk in a straight line, do not stretch your spine to the point where your head tends to tilt backward. Place your hands on your knees or in your lap.

Breathe slowly, gently, and effortlessly, without noise or jerks. Close your mouth, relax your jaw, and allow your lower and upper lips to gently touch. Rest your upper row of teeth against the lower row, but do not exert any mental effort to bring this about. Rest your tongue on the floor of your mouth, with the tip gently touching the ridge just above your upper teeth.

Now bring your attention to your breath. Breathe in and out smoothly and effortlessly. In chaturtha pranayama you pay attention only to your inhalation and exhalation. Breath retention is not part of the process but rather a naturally occurring phenomenon, which arises effortlessly. Like the previous pranayamas, chaturtha pranayama is monitored by space and time; however, this monitoring is done only during the inhalation and the exhalation, and even that disappears when a naturally occurring retention takes over.

Inhalation and exhalation have a beginning point in both time and space. When you are inhaling, there is a particular moment when you feel the touch of incoming air at the threshold of your nostrils. In this pranayama, the threshold of your nostrils is the space where your inhalation begins; time is identified by exactly when the incoming air touches that threshold. Monitoring by number is omitted because if you attempt to keep track of the number of breaths, the counting will disturb the peaceful quality of this pranayama. Within a minute or two, the mind and the breath blend into each other so perfectly that attention to time quickly fades. Therefore, in reality, this pranayama is monitored only by space, and even that quietly and effortlessly.

Be sensitive to your breathing. Mentally register the instant when the incoming breath touches the threshold of your nostrils and identify the precise spot where you feel that touch. From here, continue inhaling and allow your mind to follow the flow of the breath. Your breath travels deeper into your nostrils, passes through the space between the eyebrows, reaches all the way to the center of the forehead and far beyond. Do not imagine anything—simply let your mind feel the flow of your breath as it moves upward. Let your mind go as high and deep as your breath goes. Do not push your breath or your mind to go higher than they tend to go naturally. Then, without pausing, begin exhaling. Let your mind follow the movement of your exhalation as it travels downward, until it reaches the precise point where your inhalation began. One inhalation and exhalation constitutes one breath. Take 3 to 5 breaths.

The next step requires feeling the flow of your inhalation and exhalation closer to the ceiling of your nasal passage. The goal is to cultivate sensitivity to the movement of the subtler counterpart of your breathing in the space in front of your face, the space occupied by your frontal lobes, and the space just in front of your forehead.

Physiologically and anatomically, air travels through your nostrils in the form of breath, but here you are training your mind to sense breath as prana as it travels through the pranic field housing the entire region of your face, forehead, head, brain, and sense organs. To accomplish this, at the first instant of your inhalation, transport your awareness from the threshold of your nostrils to the tip of your nostrils. Mentally, you are now in front of your face rather than in the space inside your nostrils. Continue breathing upward just as you did before. Mentally, go as high as the breath goes. Then, without creating a pause, immediately start exhaling and come down all the way to the lowest reaches of the space in front of your face. Take 3 to 5 breaths.

Then begin the next cycle of chaturtha pranayama. Inhale and exhale as you did before, but this time pay attention to the unique experience unfolding in the space corresponding to the region in the inner corners of your eyes and between the eyebrows. This experience is joyful and captivating, especially during the inhalation. The mind tends to stop here, but also has a tendency to continue traveling upward with the breath—it is pulled between two sweet experiences. Let your mind stop for a moment to observe and embrace the sweetness filling the space corresponding to the inner corners of your eyes and between the eyebrows. The process of attending to this joyful feeling does not disturb the gentle and smooth upward flow of your inhalation.

Because the breath and the mind are accustomed to moving as one fully unified stream of awareness, the mind will identify and capture the joy of this space in an instant and resume its journey to the center of the forehead. Do not make an effort to stop your mind in this space filled with joy. And do not attempt to create this experience, nor be anxious about when and how it will arise. Do not use your imagination. When this experience is there, you cannot ignore it, and when it is not there, you cannot create it. Your job is simply to breathe in and out absolutely effortlessly, and let the mind accompany the peaceful flow of your breath. The experience of joy unique to this space will arise in your mind of its own accord.

Each time the breath and mind reach the space corresponding to the center of the forehead, your sensitivity to that space increases. You are able to feel and touch that space and you are able to identify its furthest frontier. There is a unique joy in observing that your inhalation reaches all the way to this furthest frontier—it is here that your inhalation terminates and your exhalation begins.

As you continue your practice, the experience of joy in the space corresponding to the inner corners of the eyes intensifies. In proportion to the intensity of that joy, the space in the center of your forehead becomes clear and well defined. Eventually, these two spheres blend and there is only one space covering the entire region of your eyes, inner corners of your eyes, eyebrows, center between the eyebrows, and forehead. As you continue the practice, this space expands. You feel its existence in front of your face and forehead—a uniquely lit space filled with joy. The center of this self-luminous space is the area known as *ajna chakra,* which corresponds physiologically to the inner space of the forehead.

At this stage, the awareness that you are breathing through your nostrils has faded. You are aware only that you are breathing. You are experiencing your breath as a wave of awareness moving up and down in the space just in front of your face. You are no longer aware of the movement of inhalation and exhalation, but rather of the subtle movement of consciousness in this space. The mind has stopped associating with the physical dimension of the breath (*gati abhava*) and instead is fully absorbed in the breath's subtle counterpart.

In this state of mental absorption in the subtle pranic movement, the physical dimension of breathing slows drastically. You may be taking only 3 to 5 breaths a minute and the length of both the inhalation and the exhalation is significantly reduced. According to Vyasa, this happens due to *bhumi jaya,* which means "victory over ground." This means you have attained such a high degree of effortlessness that physical activity has dropped to a minimum, along with your metabolic rate. All your limbs and organs are almost completely at rest. This restful condition extends all the way to your mitochondrial activity. The body's need for oxygen has dropped significantly; Thus the breath is almost suspended. This natural suspension of the breath is chaturtha pranayama.

Chaturtha pranayama is completely different from the pranayamas mentioned in the previous sutra and in all other texts. Unlike other pranayamas, here the suspension of the breath occurs neither before, after, nor in the midst of the inhalation and exhalation. As the body, mind, limbs, and organs relax, the need for oxygen diminishes, thus reducing the length of the inhalation and exhalation. This natural shortening of the breath bears no resemblance to shortness of breath; rather, it is the refinement of breath. In chaturtha pranayama we do not gasp for air. On the contrary, we fill our body with *vajra-samhananatva,* the body's innate capacity to heal and nourish itself from deep inside.

As we progress in our practice, we reach the pinnacle of chaturtha pranayama more quickly. For example, in the beginning stages, it may take 5 to 10 minutes before we experience the joy in the space surrounding the center between our eyebrows. After three months of consistent practice, we may experience the dawning of the uniquely lit space in front of our countenance in a few minutes. As stated earlier, the longer we observe the movement of the subtle counterpart of our breath in this space, the brighter the space becomes. The impurities hidden deep in our body and mind are destroyed in proportion to this brilliance. How this happens is the subject of the next sutra.

SUTRA 2:52

ततः क्षीयते प्रकाशावरणम् ।।५२।।

tataḥ kṣīyate prakāśāvaraṇam ॥ 52 ॥

tataḥ, then; *kṣīyate*, attentuated; *prakāśa*, light; *āvaraṇam*, veil

Then the veil over the light is attenuated.

Here Patanjali makes another bold statement: the practice of pranayama destroys the veil that hides our intrinsic luminosity. To understand this statement it is necessary to reflect on the fundamental philosophy and metaphysics of prana.

As stated earlier, inhalation and exhalation are merely the physical correlates of prana. Prana is different from the air we breathe. It is *brahma-spanda,* the pulsation of all-pervading, ever-present absolute being. It is the intrinsic intention of Ishvara. Prana is Ishvara's unalloyed, unconditional love. It has only one objective—to awaken individual souls and give them the strength and vision to seek and find ultimate freedom and lasting fulfillment. When the tender touch of prana awakens us from our deep slumber in the unfathomable darkness of death, the karmic forces that were absorbed into nothingness at the time of death instantly come back to life. They create an environment for us to be reborn. Propelled by prana, these karmic forces attract the *tanmatras,* the imperceptible subtle matter needed to form a body. Thus we are conceived (*Shiva Sutra* 1:19).

The same pranic force also awakens our mind. The instant the mind awakens, numberless samskaras begin to pulsate. Long before our brain and nervous system develop, the mind begins dreaming. As *Shiva Sutra* 2:4 tells us, the contents of these dreams have no specific cognitions. In the earliest days of gestation, our dreams are enveloped in deep darkness. In the absence of both subjective and objective awareness, the mind and the memories flashing through it are intermingled. The mind is not cognizant enough to comprehend memories as cognition. Furthermore, the memories are indistinguishable and without sequence.

As we have seen in *Yoga Sutra* 2:9, this same phenomenon arose when our consciousness was collapsing into death. By disconnecting prana from us, divine providence put a thick veil over our memories, enabling us to rest on the bed of death in an absolute lack of self-awareness. Now it arises again as consciousness takes on a new life. By again uniting us with prana, divine providence removes the veil over our memories, enabling us to regain our self-awareness, as well as all our indistinguishable non-linear memories.

As we are further infused with prana shakti, we begin to recall our past experiences in a relatively more distinguishable, linear manner. This is overwhelming for the fledging mind. The next wave of prana comes to our aid in two different ways: it infuses our mind with a greater intensity of comprehension (*jnana*), and veils the memories that serve no purpose in the life about to unfold (*Bhagavad Gita* 15:15). This veil is avidya. Because of avidya, we comprehend our self and our memories only to an extent that does not overwhelm our fledgling mind.

With the return of avidya, the other four afflictions—our shrunken sense of self-identity, attachment, aversion, and fear—also return. Instantly the principles of time, space, number, and notions of duality—such as near, far; big, small; good, bad; possible, impossible—are added to the veil of avidya.

As avidya envelops us from every direction and in every manner, we become individuals with limited power and knowledge. We are hidden from our mind, and our mind is hidden from us. We are hidden from inside as well as from outside. Avidya seeps into every nook and cranny of our mind and consciousness. It is as alive as they are. Powered by prana, the veil of avidya allows a limited number of memories to flash in our mind in a precise order. Under the sway of avidya, the mind comprehends in a limited manner. In response to this dim and fragmented comprehension, the building materials of our body—earth, water, fire, air, and space—are pulled toward the core of our being. Only after dulling the immense powers and privileges of these elements does avidya fashion them into a developing fetus. Thus we enter this world with a body and mind whose powers and privileges are significantly compromised. With this kind of body and mind we begin life's journey and struggle to find life's purpose.

As soon as the veil of avidya is destroyed, we gain access to all the powers and privileges inherent in our body and mind—we acquire our innate wisdom (*Shiva Sutra* 3:6–7). We are able to create a world of our choice in direct proportion to the thinning of this veil (SS 3:17). The attenuation of avidya comes from understanding the dynamics of prana, which breathed life into it in the first place. To do this, we must survey the size of our personal world.

According to the *Yoga Vasishtha,* our personal world encompasses the space occupied by our body and the space around our body spanning the width of 12 fingers. We are born with this much space. We exist, breathe, live, and die in this space. Our experience of pleasure and pain, satisfaction and frustration, hunger and thirst, sickness and health is confined to this space. We sit, move, sleep, dream, meditate, and attain samadhi in this space. Acquisition of this space is birth; eviction from it is death. In union with prana, we acquire this space, and with disunion we lose it.

The space allotted for our personal world is saturated with prana. This space is exclusively ours—experientially it is us. Our physical body with all its limbs and organs is suspended in this pranically charged space and anchored there by strong pranic currents. These same pranic currents anchor our organs in the space that appears to be "inside" the body.

It is important to remember that prana is the first and foremost manifestation of Ishvara's prakriti and as such is omnipresent. Prana is inside the space allotted to us as well as everywhere outside. However, from our perspective, there is a greater concentration of prana shakti in the space that houses our body and the 12-finger-width area surrounding it. Our intimate relationship with this pranic saturation enables us to be a self-contained, autonomous entity. We are a complete and independent being only because we are *prani,* "an entity infused with prana; the possessor of prana; an entity adopted by prana." Yogis describe prana as the godparent of every living being in the universe. Discovery of this perennial godparent begins with understanding our breath, the most significant and accessible physiological correlate of prana.

The practice of pranayama enables us to discover and embrace the deeper dimension of our breath. To understand how pranayama introduces us to our prana shakti and how a concentrated and incessant flow of prana eliminates our inner impurities, including the veil of avidya, we must revisit *chaturtha pranayama* and examine a facet not discussed in the previous sutra.

According to the *Yoga Vasishtha* ("Nirvana Prakarana," chapters 24–26), chaturtha pranayama has eight aspects. They are not dependent on how we inhale, exhale, and retain our breath, but rather on where we do this in the space allotted to us. There are three distinct areas: the space inside our body, the space spanning 12 finger-widths outside our body, and the space beyond.

The first two aspects of chaturtha pranayama are associated with the two distinct spaces where we inhale: in the space that stretches 12 finger-widths outside the threshold of the nostrils, and in the space stretching from the threshold of the nostrils to the center of the forehead. There are also two distinct spaces where we exhale: in the space stretching from the threshold of the nostrils to 12 finger-widths outside it, and in the space beyond this perimeter.

The remaining four aspects of chaturtha pranayama are associated with breath retention. The first two are internal kumbhaka. We inhale in the space outside the threshold of our nostrils and retain the breath there, or inhale in the space between the threshold of our nostrils and the forehead and retain the breath somewhere in that space. The remaining two aspects are external kumbhaka. We exhale in the space outside the threshold of our nostrils and retain the breath there, or exhale beyond the 12-finger-width perimeter and retain the breath there. This concept of inhalation, exhalation, and retention is highly refined, and the process is extremely precise.

Prana is subtle and so are its functions. It is everywhere inside the body and extends 12 finger-widths outside the body. But we can touch and feel its movement only in the parts of the body where its flow is significantly strong and in organs highly saturated with its intelligence. The most prominent of these are located in the space between the threshold of the nostrils and the center of the forehead.

Anatomically, when we inhale, the air enters our nostrils, passes through the trachea, and fills our lungs. As we exhale, the process is reversed. However, the nerve receptors in our nostrils, trachea, and lungs are not designed to register the sensation of touch. Olfactory nerves register different shades of odor; Thus they function as the sense of smell but not as the sense of touch. The slight sensation of touch we experience there resides in the skin covering the threshold of the nostrils. Thus when air travels in and out, we are hardly aware of it. Because we have seen the drawings of the anatomical dimensions of our breathing, we may imagine the movement of air, but we cannot actually feel it.

However, there is a strong sensation of energy-like movement from the threshold of the nostrils all the way to the forehead that has no connection with the passage of air. We are able to experience this sensation because this region is highly saturated with pranic intelligence and because the flow of prana here is significantly strong. This is one of the few regions in our body where we can clearly observe the distinction between the movement of air and the movement of prana shakti.

By manipulating the flow of our inhalation and exhalation, we can calm our nervous system and free our mind from neurological and physiological distractions to a great extent. With practice, we can then put our inhalation and exhalation on autopilot and employ our mind exclusively in observing the continuous movement of prana in this region.

As noted earlier, maturity in the practice of chaturtha pranayama results in the dawning of a brilliantly lit space in front of our countenance. It is in this space that we touch and feel the movement of prana. It is in this space that our mind embraces the pranic waves. Its timeless familiarity with prana causes the mind to fall in love with prana. The mind becomes concentrated.

As practice continues, the space in front of the face becomes more vibrant, causing the mind to become increasingly concentrated. The high degree of brilliance engendered by pranayama gives the mind the vision to see what once was beyond its comprehension. It is charged with the power to see the numberless layers of the veil of ignorance. It is also charged with the power of discernment to distinguish complex and afflicting karmic impressions from those that are simpler and less afflicting. The mind now has the courage to focus on the present and let go of the past. United with the valiant force of prana, it has the capacity to focus on anything it chooses—a subject Patanjali explores in the next sutra.

SUTRA 2:53

धारणासु च योग्यता मनसः ॥५३॥

dhāraṇāsu ca yogyatā manasaḥ ॥ 53 ॥

dhāraṇāsu, concentrations; *ca,* also; *yogyatā*, qualification; *manasaḥ*, of mind

The mind is also qualified for concentrations.

Yoga is defined as arresting and eventually transcending the mind's roaming tendencies. To achieve this objective we are advised to concentrate on a singular object. But most of us have a mind that is disturbed and scattered. Trying to concentrate on a singular object with a disturbed, distracted mind is as absurd as trying to sit on your own shoulders. We must first build the capacity to concentrate. As we saw in the previous sutra, this capacity comes from the practice of pranayama.

With the exception of *chaturtha,* the fourth pranayama, and the pranayama known as *pracchardana vidharana* (YS 1:34), all breathing exercises awaken our dormant vigor and vitality by churning the nervous system, accelerating the functions of the internal organs, and unblocking the nadis. In addition, pracchardana vidharana brings our pranic awareness to a focal point—we become acutely aware of the prana shakti in the center of the forehead. This awareness is engendered by vigorous inhalation and exhalation and is therefore accompanied by a high degree of activity. The mind can concentrate on the pranic field peacefully only after this pranic activity calms, which takes time. In chaturtha pranayama, we reach this tranquil state of pranic activity effortlessly and relatively quickly.

The simple version of chaturtha pranayama described in sutra 2:51 enables us to cultivate sensitivity to pranic movement in the region between the threshold of the nostrils and the center of the forehead. This infuses the mind with the capacity to concentrate in this region. As practice matures, the mind becomes capable of concentrating at the center of this region, which has the highest degree of pranic concentration. In the scriptures, this spot in our mental space is known as the *ajna chakra*. In other words, the simple version of chaturtha pranayama helps the mind build its capacity to concentrate at the ajna chakra. The eight types of chaturtha pranayama described in sutra 2:52 empower the mind to concentrate on any object inside or outside the body, in the present, past, or future.

In one type of chaturtha pranayama, for example, our focus is on feeling the touch of pranic movement in the space spanning 12 finger-widths outside our nostrils. This helps the mind build its capacity to concentrate on any spot within this field. With practice we can reach not only the space in front of our nostrils but the space in front of any part of our body as well. While lying on our back, for example, we can feel the pranic movement 12 finger-widths from our toes and allow our awareness to move with prana as it enters our personal space during inhalation and travels all the way to the center of the forehead and beyond. When engaged in this type of chaturtha pranayama we can choose any spot inside the body or any spot 12 finger-widths outside the body as an object of concentration.

Similarly, in another type of chaturtha pranayama, we pay attention to the movement of prana well away from the 12-finger-width perimeter around our body. With the mastery of this pranayama, the mind is charged with the capacity to focus anywhere in the outer world.

The capacity for mental concentration engendered by these pranayamas enables yogis to perform extraordinary feats—a subject which Patanjali elaborates on in detail in the third chapter of the *Yoga Sutra*. Because here, in "Sadhana Pada," Patanjali's central focus is the attenuation of afflictions and the attainment of samadhi (YS 2:2), the power of concentration is best directed toward discovering the mysteries of our own body, mind, and senses and, ultimately, accomplishing life's purpose. In this light, the power of concentration engendered by pranayama enables us to attain mastery over our senses, which otherwise continually throw the mind into states of disturbance, stupefaction, and distraction. That is the subject of the next sutra.

SUTRA 2:54

स्वविषयासम्प्रयोगे चित्तस्यस्वरूपानुकार
इवेन्द्रियाणां प्रत्याहारः ॥५४॥

svaviṣayāsamprayoge cittasyasvarūpānukāra
ivendriyāṇāṁ pratyāhāraḥ ॥ 54 ॥

sva, one's own; *viṣaya,* object; *asamprayoge,* lack of contact; *cittasya,* of mind; *svarūpa,* essential nature; *anukāraḥ,* appearance; *iva,* like; *indriyāṇāṁ,* of the senses; *pratyāhāraḥ,* withdrawing from every direction toward a focal point

Lacking contact with their respective objects, when senses assume the nature of mind it is *pratyahara.*

Pranayama leads to pratyahara. A simplistic translation is "sense withdrawal," but this is only partially correct. In practice, pratyahara involves withdrawing the mind. *Pratyahara* is composed of *prati, a,* and *hara.* Following the grammatical rules of Sanskrit, it is translated from back to front: *hara* means "to pull, to withdraw, to bring, to carry"; *a* means "from every direction in every respect"; and *prati* means "toward." Thus *pratyahara* means "pulling the mind from every direction and in every respect to a focal point." Withdrawing the mind is a purposeful and methodical process, and the process of focusing it on a given object is even more purposeful and methodical.

Before analyzing pratyahara, we need to understand the relationship between the mind and senses. They work in unison:

the mind cannot perceive an object unless it is presented to it by the senses; unless they are accompanied by the mind, the senses cannot sense an object. Our nostrils, tongue, eyes, skin, and ears are able to smell, taste, see, touch, and hear only in the presence of the mind. These organs are connected to our cortex, the physical seat of the non-physical mind. The cognitive power flowing from the cortex to these organs infuses them with the capacity to sense the objective world.

The organs themselves are not senses; rather, the power residing in them is the senses—and that power is the mind. The mind needs the sense organs. Without them, it cannot comprehend the subtle details of its cognitions. The unique design of the sense organs enables the mind to comprehend these subtle details in five broad categories. Drawing on its numberless impressions, the mind then fabricates the rest of the details. Unless the senses have laid the groundwork, the mind will not succeed in experiencing the world to its full satisfaction but will drown in the sea of abstract cognitions regarding the contentless existence of the objective world. This experience is immensely tiring and utterly fruitless. That is why the mind has invested so much of itself in the sense organs.

Once the sense organs are formed and the relationship between the mind and the brain and between the brain and the sense organs is fully established, we busy ourselves with experiencing the world. Except when we are sleeping, the sense organs and their corresponding centers in the brain are constantly at work, relentlessly consuming sensory experiences. With each experience our desires grow, so we repeat those experiences. Repetition strengthens the memories of those experiences; those memories, in turn, create deep grooves in our mind called *samskaras*. The physical correlates of the samskaras are stored in our amygdala in the form of memories; memories manifest as habits, which inspire the mind to employ the sense organs to experience the world once again. This process fuels our craving for sensory experiences and causes the mind to be overly dependent on the senses. Lacking vigilance and self-mastery, the mind chases desires and cravings, and the senses make this possible.

Every sensory pursuit takes a toll on our body, mind, and senses. The mind, working under the influence of desires, cravings, and entrenched habits, justifies its sensory pursuits. We are so smitten by sensory allurements that, for the most part, we are oblivious of the far-reaching consequences. We seek a remedy only when we find ourselves in the grip of exhaustion, and we seek it with the help of an incapacitated mind. This is where the practice of pratyahara comes in.

Pratyahara is a two-part practice: withdraw the mind from all sensory engagements and then focus it on an object that transcends the ordinary realm of the senses. Here is how it is done.

Begin by sitting in a meditative pose. Withdraw your mind from the external world—resolve to be aware only of your body and the space it occupies. By simply paying attention to your body, you will be able to withdraw your mind from all other places and concerns. While paying attention to your body, do not mentally outline it or survey your individual limbs and organs. Simply become aware of your own existence. The greater your awareness of the space related to your physical existence, the weaker your awareness will be of everything else. This is because the mind, which uses the senses to travel in the objective world, has returned to its workplace—the nostrils, tongue, eyes, skin, and ears. From these sense organs, it withdraws to its physical home base—the cortex.

The mind's journey from the objective world to the cortex

constitutes only half of the practice of pratyahara. The remaining half is accomplished by leading the mind to a state where it resumes *svarupa-anukara,* its essential nature. Awareness of its intrinsic luminosity is the mind's nature. Subtle impressions and the roaming tendencies arising from them block this intrinsic luminosity. Once the mind is disconnected from sensory objects, it has an opportunity to pay attention to its intrinsic nature. The process of attending to and becoming absorbed in its pure nature is the final step of pratyahara.

This final step consists of a methodical practice involving more than simply resolving not to be aware of the objects of the senses. As stated earlier, prana pervades every nook and cranny of our body. It is inside our body as well as 12 finger-widths outside it. There is a greater concentration of prana shakti at certain spots within this space. Each of these spots is known as a *marma-sthana,* a concentrated pranic field. The final step of pratyahara involves entering these pranic fields one by one, focusing the mind there for a while, then moving on to the next pranic field. In the context of surgery, ayurvedic texts list 107 or 108 marma-sthanas. The yoga tradition lists 28 and emphasizes only those most significant in the practice of pratyahara. The physical correlates of these significant pranic fields are the nostrils, the inner corners of the eyes, the center between the eyebrows, the forehead, the crown of the head, the heart, and the navel area.

The practice of the final step of pratyahara begins with chaturtha pranayama, as described in sutra 2:51. When you have become fully aware of your body and the space occupied by it, pay attention to your breath. Inhale and exhale gently and smoothly, without noise or jerks. As you go deeper into the practice of chaturtha pranayama, a pranically charged space emerges in front of your face. This space is intrinsically filled with profound joy and tranquility. As you allow your mind to accompany the pranic movement in this field, your breath becomes further refined.

This refinement is characterized by two factors: the number of breaths per minute drops, and the mind's roaming tendencies subside dramatically. For example, if in the normal course of life you are accustomed to taking 15 breaths per minute, at the peak of chaturtha pranayama you may be taking only 8 breaths per minute. Similarly, if you were only able to concentrate on an object for a minute, in chaturtha pranayama you are able to concentrate for two minutes or more. You are taking fewer breaths because your limbs, organs, and systems are resting deeply. Your mind is stable on an object for longer, because the senses are no longer in contact with their respective objects and, further, they are absorbed in the cortical brain. There is no awareness of smell, taste, sight, touch, or sound. The mind is so absorbed in the self-lit pranic field that it has become aware of its own inner luminosity, *jyotishmati*. This awareness is intrinsically accompanied by pure joy, *vishoka*. Luminosity has destroyed the darkness of ignorance, and joy has quelled all craving. The mind has reclaimed its innate vibrancy and joy.

Then what is the difference between chaturtha pranayama and pratyahara? Brahmananda explains this clearly in his commentary on the *Hatha Yoga Pradipika*. Referring to the *Yoga Chintamani,* he says, "The advanced stages of pranayama are known by the terms *pratyahara, dharana, dhyana,* and *samadhi*" (HYP 2:12). When we are able to hold our mind on a given object for the period of time required to take 12 normal breaths, it is defined as pranayama.

According to Brahmananda, the length of a normal breath is measured by the time it takes for a healthy person to complete one inhalation and exhalation while sleeping. While sleeping, a healthy person breathes 15 to 20 times per minute. Thus one normal breath takes 3 to 4 seconds. When the mind disconnects from its roaming tendencies and remains focused on a particular pranic field for 12 breaths, it is defined as pranayama. In other words, pranayama is characterized by our mind's ability to remain focused on prana for not less than 48 seconds. A minimum of 48 seconds is required for the bonding between prana and mind to fully mature. Thus pranayama is not defined by how long we hold the breath but rather by how long we hold our mind on the subtle movement of prana in the pranic field.

When mental concentration is 12 times longer than the period of concentration defining pranayama, it is pratyahara. In other words, when we are able to hold our mind on a marma-sthana for not less than 576 seconds (12 x 48) or 9.6 minutes, we have entered the realm of pratyahara. Dharana, concentration, is 12 times longer than pratyahara. Our capacity to concentrate increases with practice, allowing dharana to mature into dhyana and samadhi.

Describing the details of this process (HYP 2:12), Brahmananda claims that lower-grade pranayama is when we are able to stay focused on prana for a period of time required for 12 breaths (approximately 48 seconds). When concentration is extended to 84 breaths (approximately 5.6 minutes), it is medium-grade pranayama. When concentration is prolonged for 125 breaths (approximately 8.5 minutes), it is the highest-grade pranayama. We transition from this highest-grade pranayama to pratyahara as soon as our concentration stretches beyond 8.5 minutes. Remember, however, that this is an approximation of our inner experience, not a rigid formula.

According to the tradition, it takes 8 to 10 minutes for the mind to charge itself with the intrinsic vigor, vitality, strength, stamina, and endurance of prana to recognize, face, and conquer the deeply rooted samskaras which churn our mind and senses and force them to run after long-cherished habits, cravings, and addictions. This conquest is the subject of the next sutra.

SUTRA 2:55

ततः परमा वश्यतेन्द्रियाणाम् ॥५५॥

tataḥ paramā vaśyatendriyāṇām ॥ 55 ॥

tataḥ, from that; *paramā,* the highest; *vaśyatā*, mastery; *indriyāṇām*, senses

From that [pratyahara] comes the highest level of mastery over the senses.

The senses are powerful and to some extent autonomous. There are occasions when they do their job whether we want them to or not. For example, when there are loud sounds we do not want to hear, the ears sense them anyway. And, in some instances, the senses exercise their autonomy indiscriminately. For example, drug addicts know drugs are destructive and disempowering yet cannot stop from indulging. The practice of pratyahara enables us to attain mastery over these powerful and autonomous senses. This mastery is twofold: victory over the addictive behaviors of the senses, and unfoldment of their extraordinary power.

First, let us look at the dynamics of conquering the addictive behaviors of the senses. As we have seen, every action creates an impression. Impressions become strong and deep either when actions are repeated again and again, or when the intention behind them is intense. In some cases, impressions become strong when the actions are propelled by powerful forces and substances. This is what Vyasa calls *vyasana,* addiction. Addiction is a strong craving—powerful enough to crush our determination, forcing our mind and senses to engage in actions we know to be harmful.

When, with the practice of pratyahara, we withdraw our mind from sensory realms, unite it with prana, and maintain this union for more than 8 to 9 minutes, the mind becomes strong enough to recognize, face, and conquer powerful sensory cravings. Even the strongest sense cravings are weaker than our willpower and determination. With the help of this newborn willpower we can calm and eventually stop sensory turmoil. However, the rise in willpower and determination is always in proportion to the degree of perfection in pratyahara. We do not become perfect overnight. As we continue the practice, the duration of pratyahara increases. Coupled with the power of repetition, the ever-increasing duration of the practice infuses the sensory centers in the cortex with the vigor and vitality of prana, freeing them from the dominance of sensory habits.

Addictive behavior makes an impression on our sense organs and brain, as well as on our mind. As this process advances, our body chemistry is affected. By the time this process matures and causes a chemical imbalance, there is little hope of fixing it simply by summoning our willpower. The repeated and prolonged practice of pratyahara reverses this process and eventually heals the damage caused by the addictive behavior of our sense organs, brain, nervous system, and endocrine system.

The reason pratyahara reverses the addictive behavior of our senses and heals the damage it causes is simple. As part of the practice, the mind is brought back to the body from all corners of the world. Then it is led point-by-point from one *marma-sthana* to the next. This allows the mind to become familiar with the intrinsic quality of those pranic fields and develop a loving bond with them. Finally, the mind is led to the center of the forehead, where it is united with one of the most concentrated pranic fields, the *ajna chakra.*

As we repeat the practice again and again, the pranic field covering the entire space above our shoulders becomes charged with the united forces of mind and prana. The joy engendered by this union engulfs the mind's roaming tendencies. The cortex, which is the seat of *manas,* the thinking mind, stops brooding on the future. This leads to freedom from anxiety. The amygdala, which is the seat of *chitta,* the storehouse of memories, stops interacting with emotions associated with past issues. This leads to freedom from sorrow.

The space housing the cortex and the amygdala also houses other parts of the brain, such as the medulla oblongata and the pituitary gland. The medulla governs the functions of the heart, the lungs, and the diaphragm. A pranically charged medulla becomes acutely alert and starts working more efficiently. Similarly, the pituitary gland becomes more perceptive and begins to regulate the endocrine system skillfully. In general, the brain, which is the seat of all mental faculties, becomes tranquil and no longer bombards the body with false and confusing signals. We are completely at rest. In this state, the innate wisdom of the body accelerates the healing process. We are energized by prana shakti. This revitalization results in the unfoldment of the extraordinary power of our senses and mind.

Normally, we perceive objects when they are in direct contact with the senses. But as soon as the power behind the sense organs becomes established in its point of origin—the mind—we begin to comprehend objects imperceptible to our senses. This is because the entire field of our brain is energized and lit by the combined luminosity of prana and the mind. The vast information stored in the various parts of the brain is at our disposal. The mind, which is both calm and alert, is able to string together a long chain of information and use it to intuitively understand what we could not have understood with the help of the senses alone. For example, we cannot hear the sound of an exploding star, and yet with the help of a one-pointed, sharp mind, we can comprehend it and thus discover devices that enable us to experience it. Like our sense organs, these devices are tools invented by our mind. The fields of mathematics, quantum physics, and genetics, to cite only a few examples, are the work of our highly potent and perceptive mind.

This same mental capacity helps us earn the qualifications we need to discover our core being, which exists outside the domain of the mind's normal capacity. In order to comprehend the essence of the inner being, the mind has to cultivate two qualities: it must learn to turn itself inward, and it must rise above its habit of identifying things as objects of its cognition—it must transcend its habit of clinging to subject-object awareness in relation to everything it perceives. The practice of pratyahara, which is a continuation of *chaturtha pranayama*, trains the mind to cultivate these two qualities. The intrinsic joy (*vishoka*) and luminosity (*jyotishmati*) of prana shakti capture the mind so completely that it stops traveling into the external world and begins to travel toward the core of prana shakti. The joy and luminosity of prana shakti are the ever-radiating *svabhava* of Ishvara. They are the source of everything that exists, including ourselves.

Once we reach this far, the mind drops its long-cherished habit of identifying and possessing the objects of its cognition. The joy of losing itself in this highly concentrated field far exceeds the joy of maintaining subject-object awareness. At this point of realization, the mind is totally free from all fears. It spontaneously and effortlessly drops all its defenses and begins to take on the qualities of prana shakti. The mind soaks up primordial joy and luminosity. It becomes prana shakti and, as such, experiences itself as an expression of the *sankalpa* of Ishvara. The mind no longer perceives Ishvara as an object of its perception. In sutra 2:41, Vyasa describes this as *atma-darshana-yogyatva,* the qualification of having the experience of *atman*. As the Upanishads say, the knower of truth becomes truth. At the maturity of the process engendered by pratyahara, the mind dissolves (so to speak) into atman and becomes atman. In *yoga shastra,* prana shakti and atman are one and the same. And it is in this respect that the individual self is the manifestation of the divine, Ishvara.

The longer and more frequently we attend our union with prana, the more established we become in our essential nature. This mental absorption in prana shakti wipes out our *moha*—our confusion regarding who we are, where we come from, why we exist, who sustains us, and who guides us at every stage of life. We are free from doubt. This leads us to recapture our most primordial experience—the experience of being in the full embrace of the divine. The fear of losing our possessions, including the most precious one—life in the mortal world—vanishes. We are free of fear. Free of doubt and fear, the mind spontaneously surrenders to divine will. In sutra 4:34, Patanjali calls this *svarupa pratishtha,* establishment in one's essential nature. As the *Bhagavad Gita* tells us, this is when we truly hear the voice of our soul and have the capacity to heed it (BG 18:73).

As soon as we are able to hear and heed the voice of our core being, our thoughts, speech, and actions begin to resonate with the divine will. Sensing this, nature begins to resonate with our thoughts, speech, and actions; she turns into our mother and we turn into her children. This relationship is not an intellectual construct—it is completely experiential. To nurture her children, nature manifests her extraordinary powers and offers them as gifts.

This is what Patanjali describes as *siddhis* in "Vibhuti Pada," the next chapter of the *Yoga Sutra*.

Nature's ever-unfolding gifts strengthen our realization of how fortunate we are. We realize that our good fortune has its source in divine grace. We are not born through our own effort—divine grace makes all the arrangements for our birth. This is also true of our achievements—we are successful only because nature has given us an extraordinary body and a perceptive mind. These realizations fill us with a deep sense of gratitude. This is true love. The instant it dawns, pratyahara effortlessly grows into dharana, dharana into dhyana, and dhyana into samadhi.

In concluding this chapter with pratyahara, Patanjali emphasizes that dharana, dhyana, and samadhi are not possible without pratyahara. When we are fully established in the practice of pratyahara, the remaining three stages of yoga sadhana walk into our life effortlessly. Patanjali elaborates on this in the next chapter, "Vibhuti Pada."

APPENDIXES

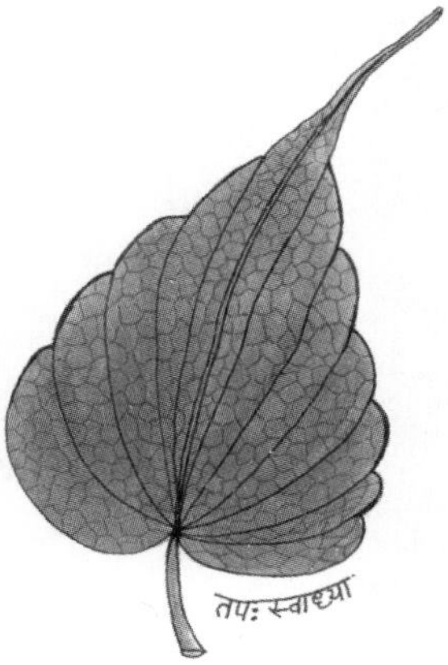

APPENDIX A

Devanagari, Transliteration, and Translation

SUTRA 2:1

तपःस्वाध्यायेश्वरप्रणिधानानि क्रियायोगः ॥१॥

tapaḥsvādhyāyeśvarapraṇidhānāni kriyāyogaḥ ‖ 1 ‖

Yoga in action is composed of austerity, self-study, and trustful surrender to Ishvara.

SUTRA 2:2

समाधिभावनार्थः क्लेशतनूकरणार्थश्च ॥२॥

samādhibhāvanārthaḥ kleśatanūkaraṇārthaśca ‖ 2 ‖

The objective of yoga is to induce samadhi and attenuate the afflictions.

SUTRA 2:3

अविद्यास्मितारागद्वेषाभिनिवेशाः क्लेशाः ।।३।।

avidyāsmitārāgadveṣābhiniveśāḥ kleśāḥ ॥ 3 ॥

Ignorance, false sense of self-identity, attachment, aversion, and fear of death are the afflictions.

SUTRA 2:4

अविद्या क्षेत्रमुत्तरेषां प्रसुप्ततनुविच्छिन्नोदाराणाम् ।।४।।

avidyā kṣetramuttareṣām prasuptatanuvicchinnodārāṇām ॥ 4 ॥

Ignorance is the ground for the remaining afflictions, whether they are dormant, attenuated, disjointed, or active.

SUTRA 2:5

अनित्याशुचिदुःखानात्मसु
नित्यशुचिसुखात्मख्यातिरविद्या ।।५।।

anityāśuciduḥkhānātmasu nityaśucisukhātmakhyātiravidyā ॥ 5 ॥

Mistaking short-lived objects, impurity, suffering, and non-being for eternity, purity, happiness, and pure being is *avidya*.

SUTRA 2:6

दृग्दर्शनशक्त्योरेकात्मतेवास्मिता ॥६॥

dṛgdarśanaśaktyorekātmatevāsmitā ॥ 6 ॥

Asmita **arises from the apparent oneness of the power of the perceiver and the power of perception.**

SUTRA 2:7

सुखानुशयी रागः ॥७॥

sukhānuśayī rāgaḥ ॥ 7 ॥

Affliction that has pleasure as its resting ground is attachment.

SUTRA 2:8

दुःखानुशयी द्वेषः ॥८॥

duḥkhānuśayī dveṣaḥ ॥ 8 ॥

Affliction that has pain as its resting ground is aversion.

SUTRA 2:9

स्वरसवाही विदुषोऽपि तथारूढोऽभिनिवेशः ॥९॥

svarasavāhī viduṣo'pi tathārūḍho'bhiniveśaḥ ॥ 9 ॥

Fear of death carries its own essence and rides [the consciousness] of even the wise.

SUTRA 2:10

ते प्रतिप्रसवहेयाः सूक्ष्माः ॥१०॥

te pratiprasavaheyāḥ sūkṣmāḥ ॥ 10 ॥

The afflictions are discarded at death only if they have become subtle.

SUTRA 2:11

ध्यानहेयास्तद्वृत्तयः ॥११॥

dhyānaheyāstadvṛttayaḥ ॥ 11 ॥

The mental tendencies associated with the afflictions can be destroyed by meditation.

SUTRA 2:12

क्लेशमूलः कर्माशयो दृष्टादृष्टजन्मवेदनीयः ॥१२॥

kleśamūlaḥ karmāśayo dṛṣṭādṛṣṭajanmavedanīyaḥ ॥ 12 ॥

The reservoir of karma is rooted in afflictions and is to be experienced in seen and unseen lives.

SUTRA 2:13

सति मूले तद्विपाको जात्यायुर्भोगाः ॥१३॥

sati mūle tadvipāko jātyāyurbhogāḥ ॥ 13 ॥

As long as the root cause [the five afflictions] persists, karmas must bear fruit, and that fruition determines our birth in a particular species, life span, and life experience.

SUTRA 2:14

ते ह्लादपरितापफलाः पुण्यापुण्यहेतुत्वात् ॥१४॥

te hlādaparitāpaphalāḥ puṇyāpuṇyahetutvāt ॥ 14 ॥

They [karmas that result in rebirth, dictate how long we live in our body, and determine our general experience] are accompanied by pleasure and pain, for they are smeared with both virtue and vice.

SUTRA 2:15

परिणामतापसंस्कारदुःखैर्गुणवृत्तिविरोधाच्च दुःखमेव सर्वं विवेकिनः ॥१५॥

pariṇāmatāpasaṁskāraduḥkhairguṇavṛttivirodhācca duḥkhameva sarvam vivekinaḥ ॥ 15 ॥

From the vantage point of a wise person, all is pain because everything is subject to change, distress, karmic impressions, and mutually contradicting forces of nature.

SUTRA 2:16

हेयं दुःखमनागतम् ॥१६॥

heyaṁ duḥkhamanāgatam ॥ 16 ॥

Pain that has not yet come can be abandoned.

SUTRA 2:17

द्रष्टृदृश्ययोः संयोगो हेयहेतुः ॥१७॥

draṣṭṛdṛśyayoḥ saṁyogo heyahetuḥ ॥ 17 ॥

The union of the seer and the seeable is the cause of pain.

SUTRA 2:18

प्रकाशक्रियास्थितिशीलं भूतेन्द्रियात्मकं भोगापवर्गार्थं दृश्यम् ॥१८॥

prakāśakriyāsthitiśīlaṁ bhūtendriyātmakaṁ
bhogāpavargārthaṁ dṛśyam ॥ 18 ॥

The objective world, composed of elements and senses and having the inherent properties of illumination, action, and stability, has a twofold purpose: fulfillment and freedom.

SUTRA 2:19

विशेषाविशेषलिङ्गमात्रालिङ्गानि गुणपर्वाणि ॥१९॥

viśeṣāviśeṣaliṅgamātrāliṅgāni guṇaparvāṇi ॥ 19 ॥

The total range of the gunas is divided into four categories: specific, unspecific, barely describable, and absolutely indescribable.

SUTRA 2:20

द्रष्टा दृशिमात्रः शुद्धोऽपि प्रत्ययानुपश्यः ॥२०॥

draṣṭā dṛśimātraḥ śuddho'pi pratyayānupaśyaḥ ॥ 20 ॥

The sheer power of seeing is the seer. It is pure, and yet it sees only what the mind shows it.

SUTRA 2:21

तदर्थ एव दृश्यस्यात्मा ॥२१॥

tadartha eva dṛśyasyātmā ॥ 21 ॥

The soul of the objective world [buddhi] is meant for purusha.

SUTRA 2:22

कृतार्थं प्रति नष्टमप्यनष्टं तदन्यसाधारणत्वात् ।।२२।।

kṛtārthaṁ prati naṣṭamapyanaṣṭaṁ tadanyasādhāraṇatvāt ॥ 22 ॥

In relation to the one whose purpose is fulfilled, the objective world is destroyed, but in relation to others it is not destroyed, for the objective world is common to all purushas.

SUTRA 2:23

स्वस्वामिशक्त्योः स्वरूपोपलब्धिहेतुः संयोगः ।।२३।।

svasvāmiśaktyoḥ svarūpopalabdhihetuḥ saṁyogaḥ ॥ 23 ॥

The union of our shakti and the shakti of Ishvara is the means of experiencing our essential nature.

SUTRA 2:24

तस्य हेतुरविद्या ।।२४।।

tasya heturavidyā ॥ 24 ॥

The cause of that [union] is ignorance.

SUTRA 2:25

तदभावात् संयोगाभावो हानं तद्दृशेः कैवल्यम् ।।२५।।

tadabhāvāt saṁyogābhāvo hānaṁ taddṛśeḥ kaivalyam ॥ 25 ॥

From the absence of that [avidya] comes the absence of mingling [of consciousness with "our" mind]. That is freedom, the absolute state of the power of seeing.

SUTRA 2:26

विवेकख्यातिरविप्लवा हानोपायः ।।२६।।

vivekakhyātiraviplavā hānopāyaḥ ॥ 26 ॥

Unshakeable discerning knowledge is the means of nullifying the misery resulting from the avidya-driven union of purusha and prakriti.

SUTRA 2:27

तस्य सप्तधा प्रान्तभूमिः प्रज्ञा ।।२७।।

tasya saptadhā prāntabhūmiḥ prajñā ॥ 27 ॥

His discerning knowledge has seven spheres; the furthest frontier is *prajna*.

SUTRA 2:28

योगाङ्गानुष्ठानादशुद्धिक्षये ज्ञानदीप्तिराविवेकख्यातेः ॥२८॥

yogāṅgānuṣṭhānādaśuddhikṣaye jñānadīptirāvivekakhyāteḥ ॥ 28 ॥

The practice of the limbs of yoga destroys impurities; thereafter, knowledge continues to brighten all the way to *viveka khyati*, the domain of unshakeable discernment.

SUTRA 2:29

यमनियमासनप्राणायामप्रत्याहारधारणाध्यान समाधयोऽष्टावङ्गानि ॥२९॥

yamaniyamāsanaprāṇāyāmapratyāhāradhāraṇādhyāna-samādhayo'ṣṭāvaṅgāni ॥ 29 ॥

Restraint, observance, physical posture, mastery of the pranic force, recalling the senses, concentration, meditation, and spiritual absorption are the eight components of yoga.

SUTRA 2:30

अहिंसासत्यास्तेयब्रह्मचर्यापरिग्रहा यमाः ॥३०॥

ahiṁsāsatyāsteyabrahmacaryāparigrahā yamāḥ ॥ 30 ॥

Non-violence, truthfulness, non-stealing, continence, and non-possessiveness are the restraints.

SUTRA 2:31

जातिदेशकालसमयानवच्छिन्नाः सार्वभौमा महाव्रतम्
॥३१॥

jātideśakālasamayānavacchinnāḥ sārvabhaumā mahāvratam
॥ 31 ॥

[The aforesaid five restraints] are not affected by the factors of class, place, time, and circumstance. They are universally applicable and constitute the great vow.

SUTRA 2:32

शौचसंतोषतपःस्वाध्यायेश्वरप्रणिधानानि नियमाः
॥३२॥

śaucasantoṣatapaḥsvādhyāyeśvarapraṇidhānāni niyamāḥ ॥ 32 ॥

Purity, contentment, austerity, self-study, and trustful surrender to Ishvara are the observances.

SUTRA 2:33

वितर्कबाधने प्रतिपक्षभावनम् ॥३३॥

vitarkabādhane pratipakṣabhāvanam ॥ 33 ॥

To arrest afflicting thoughts, cultivate thoughts opposed to them.

SUTRA 2:34

वितर्का हिंसादयः कृतकारितानुमोदिता
लोभक्रोधमोहपूर्वका मृदुमध्याधिमात्रा
दुःखाज्ञानानन्तफला इति प्रतिपक्षभावनम् ॥३४॥

vitarkā hiṁsādayaḥ kṛtakāritānumoditā
lobhakrodhamohapūrvakā mṛdumadhyādhimātrā
duḥkhājñānānantaphalā iti pratipakṣabhāvanam ॥ 34 ॥

Violence and the others are afflicting thoughts. We put these thoughts into action by ourselves, through others, or by tacit consent. These thoughts are propelled by greed, anger, or confusion. They are mild, intermediate, or intense. We nullify these afflicting thoughts by realizing they bear unending fruit of pain and ignorance.

SUTRA 2:35

अहिंसाप्रतिष्ठायां तत्सन्निधौ वैरत्यागः ॥३५॥

ahiṁsāpratiṣṭhāyāṁ tatsannidhau vairatyāgaḥ ॥ 35 ॥

In the company of a yogi established in non-violence, animosity vanishes.

SUTRA 2:36

सत्यप्रतिष्ठायां क्रियाफलाश्रयत्वम् ।।३६।।

satyapratiṣṭhāyāṁ kriyāphalāśrayatvam ‖ 36 ‖

When a yogi is established in truthfulness, actions begin to bear fruit.

SUTRA 2:37

अस्तेयप्रतिष्ठायां सर्वरत्नोपस्थानम् ।।३७।।

asteyapratiṣṭhāyāṁ sarvaratnopasthānam ‖ 37 ‖

When a yogi is established in non-stealing, all gems manifest.

SUTRA 2:38

ब्रह्मचर्यप्रतिष्ठायां वीर्यलाभः ।।३८।।

brahmacaryapratiṣṭhāyāṁ vīryalābhaḥ ‖ 38 ‖

A yogi established in continence gains *virya*, the capacity to transmit knowledge.

SUTRA 2:39

अपरिग्रहस्थैर्ये जन्मकथंतासम्बोधः ।।३९।।

aparigrahasthairye janmakathantāsambodhaḥ ‖ 39 ‖

With firmness in non-possessiveness comes complete understanding of the "why-ness" of birth.

SUTRA 2:40

शौचात् स्वाङ्गजुगुप्सा परैरसंसर्गः ॥४०॥

śaucāt svāṅgajugupsā parairasaṁsargaḥ ॥ 40 ॥

From purity arises sensitivity to the unclean nature of one's own body; [that leads to] unmixing with others.

SUTRA 2:41

सत्त्वशुद्धिसौमनस्यैकाग्र्येन्द्रियजयात्मदर्शनयोग्यत्वानि च ॥४१॥

sattvaśuddhisaumanasyaikāgryendriyajayātmadarśanayog-yatvāni ca ॥ 41 ॥

[From purity arises] the purity of our essential being, a positive mind, one-pointedness, victory over the senses, and the qualification for having direct experience of our self.

SUTRA 2:42

संतोषादनुत्तमः सुखलाभः ॥४२॥

santoṣādanuttamaḥ sukhalābhaḥ ॥ 42 ॥

From contentment comes happiness without equal.

SUTRA 2:43

कायेन्द्रियसिद्धिरशुद्धिक्षयात् तपसः ।।४३।।

kāyendriyasiddhiraśuddhikṣayāt tapasaḥ ॥ 43 ॥

Austerity destroys impurities. From that come yogic accomplishments pertaining to the body and senses.

SUTRA 2:44

स्वाध्यायादिष्टदेवतासम्प्रयोगः ।।४४।।

svādhyāyādiṣṭadevatāsamprayogaḥ ॥ 44 ॥

From self-study comes the opportunity to be in the company of bright beings [of our choice].

SUTRA 2:45

समाधिसिद्धिरीश्वरप्रणिधानात् ।।४५।।

samādhisiddhirīśvarapraṇidhānāt ॥ 45 ॥

From trustful surrender to Ishvara comes samadhi.

SUTRA 2:46

स्थिरसुखम् आसनम् ।।४६।।

sthirasukham āsanam ॥ 46 ॥

A stable and comfortable posture is *asana*.

SUTRA 2:47

प्रयत्नशैथिल्यानन्तसमापत्तिभ्याम् ॥४७॥

prayatnaśaithilyānantasamāpattibhyām ॥ 47 ॥

[Perfection in asana is attained] by loosening of [tension caused by] effort and by [mental] absorption in the infinite.

SUTRA 2:48

ततो द्वन्द्वानभिघातः ॥४८॥

tato dvandvānabhighātaḥ ॥ 48 ॥

From that [comes] lack of injury caused by the pairs of opposites.

SUTRA 2:49

तस्मिन्सति श्वासप्रश्वासयोर्गतिविच्छेदः प्राणायामः ॥४९॥

tasminsati śvāsapraśvāsayorgativicchedaḥ prāṇāyāmaḥ ॥ 49 ॥

Complete mastery over the roaming tendencies of inhalation and exhalation is *pranayama*; it is to be practiced only after mastering asana.

SUTRA 2:50

बाह्याभ्यन्तरस्तम्भवृत्तिर्देशकालसंख्याभिः परिदृष्टो दीर्घसूक्ष्मः ॥५०॥

bāhyābhyantarastambhavṛttirdeśakālasaṁkhyābhiḥ paridṛṣṭo dīrghasūkṣmaḥ ॥ 50 ॥

[Pranayama with breath retention could be] threefold: external, internal, or stopping the breath wherever it is. Each is monitored by space, time, and number, and each is characterized by its length and subtlety.

SUTRA 2:51

बाह्याभ्यन्तरविषयाक्षेपी चतुर्थः ॥५१॥

bāhyābhyantaraviṣayākṣepī caturthaḥ ॥ 51 ॥

The fourth pranayama transcends the domain of external and internal pranayamas.

SUTRA 2:52

ततः क्षीयते प्रकाशावरणम् ॥५२॥

tataḥ kṣīyate prakāśāvaraṇam ॥ 52 ॥

Then the veil over the light is attenuated.

SUTRA 2:53

धारणासु च योग्यता मनसः ॥५३॥

dhāraṇāsu ca yogyatā manasaḥ ॥ 53 ॥

The mind is also qualified for concentrations.

SUTRA 2:54

स्वविषयासम्प्रयोगे चित्तस्यस्वरूपानुकार इवेन्द्रियाणां प्रत्याहारः ॥५४॥

svaviṣayāsamprayoge cittasyasvarūpānukāra ivendriyāṇāṁ pratyāhāraḥ ॥ 54 ॥

Lacking contact with their respective objects, when senses assume the nature of mind it is *pratyahara*.

SUTRA 2:55

ततः परमा वश्यतेन्द्रियाणाम् ॥५५॥

tataḥ paramā vaśyatendriyāṇām ॥ 55 ॥

From that [pratyahara] comes the highest level of mastery over the senses.

APPENDIX B

Detailed Translation (Word by Word)

SUTRA 2:1

तपःस्वाध्यायेश्वरप्रणिधानानि क्रियायोगः ॥१॥

tapaḥ-svādhyāya-īśvara-praṇidhānāni kriyā-yogaḥ ॥ 1 ॥

Yoga in action is composed of austerity, self-study, and trustful surrender to Ishvara.

tapaḥ- *nom. sg. n.* austerity; heat; a discipline or observance to cleanse the body and purify the mind; a spiritual practice to transcend our physical and mental limitations. As a verb, it means "to heat; to glow; to shine; to purify; to fire; to change; to transform."

sva-adhyāya- self study; self-reflection grounded in an understanding of inner reality

sva, self; one's own; pertaining to inner reality; *adhyāya,* grounded in understanding; having knowledge as its core *īśvara-praṇidhānāni*

nom. pl. n. trustful surrender to *īśvara*; complete faith in the guiding and protecting power of the absolute reality

īśvara, guiding and protecting force; the omniscient, primordial being; the teacher of all previous teachers; the soul free of all afflictions, karmas, and fruits of karmas; *praṇidhāna,* trustful surrender; complete recognition; embracing tightly; keeping at the center of life

kriyā-yogaḥ *nom. sg. m.* yoga in action; the yoga that can be practiced even by those with a somewhat unsteady mind

kriyā, action; effort; to initiate; to move with purpose and goal; *yoga,* the process of acquiring a calm and tranquil mind

SUTRA 2:2

समाधिभावनार्थः क्लेशतनूकरणार्थश्च ।।२।।

samādhi-bhāvana-arthaḥ kleśa-tanūkaraṇa-arthaḥ ca ॥ 2 ॥

The objective of yoga is to induce samadhi and attenuate the afflictions.

samādhi-bhāvana-arthaḥ

nom. sg. m. to induce a state of total mental stillness

samādhi, a completely still state of mind; the highest state of spiritual absorption; *bhāvana,* notion; to induce; to make happen; *artha,* objective; meaning

kleśa-tanūkaraṇa-arthaḥ

nom. sg. m. with the objective of minimizing the source of the afflictions

kleśa, affliction; the source of all pains and miseries; the source of bondage; *tanūkaraṇa,* the process of eliminating; minimization; to weaken; *artha,* meaning; objective; goal

ca and

SUTRA 2:3

अविद्यास्मितारागद्वेषाभिनिवेशाः क्लेशाः ।।३।।

avidyā-asmitā-rāga-dveṣa-abhiniveśāḥ kleśāḥ ॥ 3 ॥

Ignorance, false sense of self-identity, attachment, aversion, and fear of death are the afflictions.

avidyā- ignorance; lack of understanding; incorrect understanding; belief in that which is contrary to truth; mistaking the unreal for the real

asmitā- I-am-ness; false sense of self-identity; limited sense of being; I-am-ness confined by time and space; self-individuation; experiencing oneself in isolation from one's fullness

rāga- attachment; coloring; attraction to what is colored with prejudice and preoccupation; the binding force of desire; lust for charms and temptations of the world; holding onto what appears to be pleasant; the mind's inability to let go

dveṣa- aversion; hatred

abhi-ni-veśāḥ	*nom. pl. m.* that which has entered or penetrated our entire being completely and from every direction; fear of losing life; fear of death *abhi,* from every direction; in every respect; *ni,* completely; *veśa,* piercing; penetrating; drilling
kleśāḥ	*nom. pl. m.* afflictions; that which painfully pierces every aspect of our being

SUTRA 2:4

अविद्या क्षेत्रमुत्तरेषां प्रसुप्ततनुविच्छिन्नोदाराणाम् ॥४॥

avidyā kṣetram uttareṣām prasupta-tanu-vicchinna-udārāṇām ॥ 4 ॥

Ignorance is the ground for the remaining afflictions, whether they are dormant, attenuated, disjointed, or active.

avidyā	*nom. sg. f.* ignorance; lack of understanding; incorrect understanding; belief in that which is contrary to truth; mistaking the unreal for the real
kṣetram	*nom. sg. n.* field; farmland; ground; locus; starting point; origin
uttareṣām	*gen. pl. m.* of *uttara,* proceeding; upcoming; next
prasupta-	dormant
tanu-	attenuated; feeble; weak; thin; barely alive
vicchinna-	disjointed; broken; frequently interrupted
udārāṇām	*gen. pl. m.* of *udāra,* generous; active; full-blown

SUTRA 2:5

अनित्याशुचिदुःखानात्मसु
नित्यशुचिसुखात्मख्यातिरविद्या ॥५॥

anitya-aśuci-duḥkha-anātmasu nitya-śuci-sukha-ātmakhyātiḥ avidyā ‖ 5 ‖

Mistaking short-lived objects, impurity, suffering, and non-being for eternity, purity, happiness, and pure being is *avidya*.

anitya-	non-eternal; short-lived; mortal; ever-changing
aśuci-	impure; unclean
duḥkha-	suffering; pain; misery
anātmasu	*loc. sg. m.* of *anātman,* non-being; different from soul; different from consciousness
nitya-	eternal; everlasting; immortal
śuci-	pure; clean; unalloyed
sukha-	happiness; bliss
ātma-khyātiḥ	*nom. sg. f.* the experience of or feeling of *ātman* *ātma,* soul; consciousness; the eternal within us; *khyāti,* experience; realization
avidyā	*nom. sg. f.* ignorance; false understanding; incorrect understanding; belief in that which is contrary to truth; mistaking the unreal for the real

SUTRA 2:6

दृग्दर्शनशक्त्योरेकात्मतेवास्मिता ॥६॥

dṛk-darśana-śaktyoḥ eka-ātmatā iva asmitā ‖ 6 ‖

***Asmita* arises from the apparent oneness of the power of the perceiver and the power of perception.**

dṛk-	perceiver; seer; consciousness; *puruṣa*
darśana-	power of being perceptible; perception; seeing; sight
śaktyoḥ	*gen. du. f.* of *śakti,* power; inherent capacity
eka-ātmatā	*nom. sg. f.* apparent oneness of; false comingling of two; giving an appearance of two being one *eka,* one; *ātmatā,* self
iva	like
asmitā	*nom. sg. f.* false sense of self-identity; I-am-ness; limited sense of being

SUTRA 2:7

सुखानुशयी रागः ॥७॥

sukha-anuśayī rāgaḥ ‖ 7 ‖

Affliction that has pleasure as its resting ground is attachment.

sukha-	pleasure
anu-śayī	*nom. sg. m.* that which rests in; that which resides in *anu,* that which follows; *śayī* is derived from the verb root *śī,* to sleep; to reside in
rāgaḥ	*nom. sg. m.* attachment; coloring; attraction to what is colored

SUTRA 2:8

दुःखानुशयी द्वेषः ॥८॥

duḥkha-anuśayī dveṣaḥ ॥ 8 ॥

Affliction that has pain as its resting ground is aversion.

duḥkha- pain; sorrow

anu-śayī *nom. sg. m.* that which rests in; that which resides in

anu, that which follows; *śayī* is derived from the verb root *śī,* to rest; to sleep; to reside in

dveṣaḥ *nom. sg. m.* hatred; aversion; anger; destructive thought

SUTRA 2:9

स्वरसवाही विदुषोऽपि तथारूढोऽभिनिवेशः ॥९॥

svarasa-vāhī viduṣaḥ api tathā-rūḍhaḥ abhiniveśaḥ ॥ 9 ॥

Fear of death carries its own essence and rides [the consciousness] of even the wise.

sva-rasa-vāhī *nom. sg. m.* that which carries its own essence; that which carries its own subtle memories

sva, one's own; *rasa*, essence; flavor; juice; *vāhī,* the one who carries

viduṣaḥ *gen. sg. m.* of *vidvat,* knowledgeable; a learned person; a wise person

api even

tathā-rūḍhaḥ *nom. sg. m.* riding in that manner
tathā, in that manner; *rūḍha,* that which is riding; that which presides over

abhi-ni-veśaḥ *nom. sg. m.* that which penetrates completely from every direction and in every manner; fear of losing life; fear of death
abhi, from every direction; in every respect; *ni,* completely; *veśa,* piercing; penetrating; drilling

SUTRA 2:10

ते प्रतिप्रसवहेयाः सूक्ष्माः ॥१०॥

te prati-prasava-heyāḥ sūkṣmāḥ ॥ 10 ॥

The afflictions are discarded at death only if they have become subtle.

te they

prati-prasava-heyāḥ
nom. pl. m. of *prati-prasava-heya,* that which is discarded, abandoned, at death or after death; *prati-prasava,* death; other side of birth; opposed to birth; away from birth; dissolution
prati, prefix meaning against; as opposed to; contrary to; away from; *prasava,* birth; creation; *heya,* that which has ceased to exist; destroyed; no longer effective

sūkṣmāḥ *nom. pl. m.* of *sūkṣma,* subtle; the affliction that is transformed into *shakti mātra,* sheer power; that which is dissolved into primordial nature, *prakṛti*

SUTRA 2:11

ध्यानहेयास्तद्वृत्तयः ॥११॥

dhyāna-heyāḥ tat vṛttayaḥ ॥ 11 ॥

The mental tendencies associated with the afflictions can be destroyed by meditation.

dhyāna-	meditation
heyāḥ	*nom. pl. m.* of *heya*, to be destroyed by; to be avoided
tat	that
vṛttayaḥ	*nom. pl. f.* of *vṛtti,* mental tendency; thought construct; roaming tendency; mental modification; churning of mind

SUTRA 2:12

क्लेशमूलः कर्माशयो दृष्टादृष्टजन्मवेदनीयः ॥१२॥

kleśamūlaḥ karmāśayaḥ dṛṣṭa-adṛṣṭa-janma-vedanīyaḥ ॥ 12 ॥

The reservoir of karma is rooted in afflictions and is to be experienced in seen and unseen lives.

kleśa-mūlaḥ	*nom. sg. m.* that which has its roots in affliction *kleśa,* affliction; the fivefold affliction; *mūla,* root; ground; foundation
karma-āśayaḥ	*nom. sg. m.* the reservoir of karma *karma,* action; subtle impression of actions; *āśaya,* resting ground; container; sack; organ

dṛṣṭa-adṛṣṭa-janma-vedanīyaḥ

nom. sg. m. that which is experienced in seen and unseen lives; that which manifests in current or future lives

dṛṣṭa, seen; visible; perceptible; present; *adṛṣṭa,* unseen; invisible; imperceptible; future; *janma,* birth; *vedanīya,* to be experienced

SUTRA 2:13

सति मूले तद्विपाको जात्यायुर्भोगाः ॥१३॥

sati mūle tat vipākaḥ jāti-āyur-bhogāḥ ॥ 13 ॥

As long as the root cause [the five afflictions] persists, karmas must bear fruit, and that fruition determines our birth in a particular species, life span, and life experience.

sati	*loc. sg. m.* in the presence of; under the prevailing condition
mūle	*loc. sg. m.* of *mūla,* root; cause
tat	that
vipākaḥ	*nom. sg. m.* fruition; the condition of bearing fruit; ripening
jāti-	species
āyur-	derived from *ayus,* life span
bhogāḥ	*nom. pl. m.* experience; overall experience of life; unavoidable conditions of life

SUTRA 2:14

ते ह्लादपरितापफलाः पुण्यापुण्यहेतुत्वात् ॥१४॥

te hlāda-paritāpa-phalāḥ puṇya-apuṇya-hetutvāt ॥ 14 ॥

They [karmas that result in rebirth, dictate how long we live in our body, and determine our general experience] are accompanied by pleasure and pain, for they are smeared with both virtue and vice.

te — *nom. pl. m.* they

hlāda-paritāpa-phalāḥ
nom. pl. m. one whose overall effect is a mixture of pleasure and pain, joy and sorrow
hlāda, pleasant; joyful; favorable; *paritāpa*, condition of being scorched from every direction; pain; sorrow; *phala*, fruit

puṇya-apuṇya-hetutvāt
abl. sg. n. due to the fact that merits and demerits are the actual cause
puṇya, virtue; merit; spiritually uplifting actions; *apuṇya*, vice; spiritually degrading actions; *hetutvāt*, due to being the cause

SUTRA 2:15

परिणामतापसंस्कारदुःखैर्गुणवृत्तिविरोधाच्च दुःखमेव सर्वं विवेकिनः ॥१५॥

pariṇāma-tāpa-saṁskāra-duḥkhaiḥ guṇa-vṛtti-virodhāt ca duḥkham eva sarvam vivekinaḥ ॥ 15 ॥

From the vantage point of a wise person, all is pain because everything is subject to change, distress, karmic impressions, and mutually contradicting forces of nature.

pariṇāma-	change; effect
tāpa-	distress; heat; fever; feeling of being burnt
saṁskāra-	subtle karmic impression
duḥkhaiḥ	*ins. pl. m.* of *duḥkha,* pain resulting from change, distress, karmic impressions
guṇa-	intrinsic attribute of primordial nature; nature's three intrinsic forces, *sattva*, *rajas*, and *tamas*
vṛtti-	that which revolves; motion; modification; thought construct
virodhāt	*abl. sg. m.* of *virodha,* contradiction; opposition
ca	and; also
duḥkham	*nom. sg. m.* pain; sorrow
eva	definitely; invariably
sarvam	*nom. sg. n.* everything; all
vivekinaḥ	*abl. sg. m.* a wise person; a person endowed with the power of discernment

SUTRA 2:16

हेयं दुःखमनागतम् ॥१६॥

heyaṁ duḥkham anāgatam ॥ 16 ॥

Pain that has not yet come can be abandoned.

heyaṁ *nom. sg. m.* that which can be abandoned or renounced; that which is of an inferior nature; that which does not deserve to be entertained

duḥkham *nom. sg. m.* pain; sorrow; grief

anāgatam *nom. sg. m.* that which has not yet come

SUTRA 2:17

द्रष्टृदृश्ययोः संयोगो हेयहेतुः ॥१७॥

draṣṭṛ-dṛśyayoḥ saṁyogaḥ heya-hetuḥ ॥ 17 ॥

The union of the seer and the seeable is the cause of pain.

draṣṭṛ- seer; perceiver; consciousness; *puruṣa*; soul

dṛśyayoḥ *gen. du. m.* of *dṛśya,* perceivable; seen; the objects of perception; the objects of the senses; worldly objects

saṁyogaḥ *nom. sg. m.* complete union; complete identification

heya-hetuḥ *nom. sg. m.* cause of the avoidable; cause of that which is undesirable; cause of sorrow and pain
heya, avoidable; undesirable; *hetuḥ,* cause

SUTRA 2:18

प्रकाशक्रियास्थितिशीलं भूतेन्द्रियात्मकं भोगापवर्गार्थं दृश्यम् ॥१८॥

prakāśa-kriyā-sthiti-śīlaṁ bhūta-indriya-ātmakaṁ bhoga-apavarga-arthaṁ dṛśyam ‖ 18 ‖

The objective world, composed of elements and senses and having the inherent properties of illumination, action, and stability, has a twofold purpose: fulfillment and freedom.

prakāśa-kriyā-sthiti-śīlaṁ

nom. sg. m. having the nature of illumination, activity, and stability

prakāśa, illumination; revelation; light; understanding; the quality of *sattva*; *kriyā,* activity; action; the principle of motion; pulsation; the quality of *rajas*; *sthiti,* stability; heaviness; darkness; denseness; inertia; the quality of *tamas*; *śīlaṁ,* having the nature of

bhūta-indriya-ātmakaṁ

nom. sg. m. composed of the elements and senses

bhūta, the gross elements; *indriya,* the senses; *ātmakaṁ*, having the nature of; composed of

bhoga-apavarga-arthaṁ

nom. sg. m. the purpose of fulfillment and freedom

bhoga, fulfillment; enjoyment; experience; *apavarga,* freedom; salvation; *arthaṁ,* purpose; goal

dṛśyam *nom. sg. m.* of *dṛśya,* objective world; perceivable; knowable; comprehensible

SUTRA 2:19

विशेषाविशेषलिङ्गमात्रालिङ्गानि गुणपर्वाणि ।।१९।।

viśeṣa-aviśeṣa-liṅgamātra-aliṅgāni guṇa-parvāṇi ॥ 19 ॥

The total range of the gunas is divided into four categories: specific, unspecific, barely describable, and absolutely indescribable.

viśeṣa-	specific; distinct; discrete substance that no longer evolves into another substance
aviśeṣa-	unspecific; indistinct; substance that has evolved from a cause and serves as a cause for the evolution of another substance
liṅgamātra-	barely describable; barely comprehensible; that which can be understood through signs; that which can be hinted at; that which hints at the existence of an absolutely indescribable reality
aliṅgāni	*nom. pl. n.* of *aliṅga,* absolutely indescribable; beyond all signs and symbols
guṇa-	*sattva*, *rajas*, and *tamas*, the intrinsic attributes of *prakṛti*
parvāṇi	*nom. pl. n.* of *parva,* category; node; knot

SUTRA 2:20

द्रष्टा दृशिमात्रः शुद्धोऽपि प्रत्ययानुपश्यः ॥२०॥

draṣṭā dṛśimātraḥ śuddhaḥ api pratyaya-anupaśyaḥ ‖ 20 ‖

The sheer power of seeing is the seer. It is pure, and yet it sees only what the mind shows it.

draṣṭā *nom. sg. m.* seer

dṛśimātraḥ *nom. sg. m.* the sheer power of seeing

śuddhaḥ *nom. sg. m.* pure; unalloyed

api even; though; yet

pratyaya-anupaśyaḥ

nom. sg. m. one who sees only what is being shown by *buddhi*; one who sees through the lens of cognition; one whose comprehension follows cognition; one whose comprehension is dependent on cognition; one who no longer sees itself as the seeing power and instead perceives itself as an object of mental cognition

pratyaya, cognition; objective awareness; comprehension qualified by the sense of being an object; *anupaśya,* one who is seen as what is presented through cognition

SUTRA 2:21

तदर्थ एव दृश्यस्यात्मा ॥२१॥

tat arthaḥ eva dṛśyasya ātmā ॥ 21 ॥

The soul of the objective world [buddhi] is meant for purusha.

tat	that; seer; consciousness; consciousness fallen in the cycle of *saṁsāra; jiva,* individual self
arthaḥ	*nom. sg. m.* purpose
eva	only; precisely
dṛśyasya	*gen. sg. m.* of *dṛśya,* the objective world; worldly objects and the experiences pertaining to them
ātmā	*nom. sg. m.* soul; self; core; essence

SUTRA 2:22

कृतार्थं प्रति नष्टमप्यनष्टं तदन्यसाधारणत्वात् ॥२२॥

kṛtārthaṁ prati naṣṭam api anaṣṭaṁ tat anya-sādhāraṇatvāt ॥ 22 ॥

In relation to the one whose purpose is fulfilled, the objective world is destroyed, but in relation to others it is not destroyed, for the objective world is common to all purushas.

kṛtārthaṁ	*acc. sg. m.* of *kṛtārtha,* the one whose purpose is fulfilled *kṛta,* done; accomplished; finished; *artha,* purpose; goal; aim
prati	toward; for

naṣṭam	*acc. sg. m.* destroyed; finished; brought to a complete halt
api	yet; also; even
anaṣṭaṁ	*acc. sg. m.* not destroyed; not finished; not brought to a complete halt
tat	that
anya-	other
sādhāraṇatvāt	*abl. sg. n.* for the reason of being common

SUTRA 2:23

स्वस्वामिशक्त्योः स्वरूपोपलब्धिहेतुः संयोगः ।।२३।।

sva-svāmi-śaktyoḥ svarūpa-upalabdhi-hetuḥ saṁyogaḥ ॥ 23 ॥

The union of our shakti and the shakti of Ishvara is the means of experiencing our essential nature.

sva-	one's own; the objective world
svāmi-	*īśvara*; the master of the objective world
śaktyoḥ	*gen.du. f.* of *śakti,* power
svarūpa-	one's essential nature
upalabdhi-	achievement; realization; *darśana*
hetuḥ	*nom. sg. m.* means; cause
saṁyogaḥ	*nom. sg. m.* union; complete union; conjunction

SUTRA 2:24

तस्य हेतुरविद्या ॥२४॥

tasya hetuḥ avidyā ॥ 24 ॥

The cause of that [union] is ignorance.

tasya *gen. sg. m.* of *tat,* that

hetuḥ *nom. sg. m.* cause

avidyā *nom. sg. f.* ignorance

SUTRA 2:25

तदभावात् संयोगाभावो हानं तद्दृशेः कैवल्यम् ॥२५॥

tat abhāvāt saṁyoga-abhāvaḥ hānaṁ tat dṛśeḥ kaivalyam ॥ 25 ॥

From the absence of that [avidya] comes the absence of mingling [of consciousness with "our" mind]. That is freedom, the absolute state of the power of seeing.

tat that

abhāvāt *abl. sg. m.* of *abhāva,* absence; non-existence

saṁyoga-abhāvaḥ
nom. sg. m. absence of union; complete absence of union
saṁyoga, complete union; *abhāva*, absence; non-existence

hānaṁ *nom. sg. n.* freedom; the state free from sorrow; avoidance; nullification

tat that

dṛśeḥ *gen. sg. f.* of *dṛśi,* the seeing power of the seer

kaivalyam	*nom. sg. n.* absolute state; state of consciousness free from all conditioning	

SUTRA 2:26

विवेकख्यातिरविप्लवा हानोपायः ॥२६॥

vivekakhyātiḥ aviplavā hāna-upāyaḥ ॥ 26 ॥

Unshakeable discerning knowledge is the means of nullifying the misery resulting from the avidya-driven union of purusha and prakriti.

vivekakhyātiḥ	*nom. sg. f.* the dawning of discernment; the rise of the power of discrimination
aviplavā	*nom. sg. f.* unshakeable; that which cannot be washed away; that which cannot succumb to chaos
hāna-upāyaḥ	*nom. sg. m.* the means of nullifying sorrow *hāna,* nullification; avoidance; the state free from sorrow; liberation; *upāya,* means

SUTRA 2:27

तस्य सप्तधा प्रान्तभूमिः प्रज्ञा ॥२७॥

tasya saptadhā prāntabhūmiḥ prajñā ॥ 27 ॥

His discerning knowledge has seven spheres; the furthest frontier is *prajna*.

tasya	*gen. sg. m.* of *tat,* he; the yogi who has attained *vivekakhyati,* the power of discernment

saptadhā sevenfold; with seven distinct tiers or spheres

prānta-bhūmiḥ
nom. sg. f. the furthest frontier of *vivekakhyati*; the state beyond which there is no cognitive knowledge; knowledge par excellence
prānta, the final frontier; the extreme limit; *bhūmi*, ground

prajñā *nom. sg. f.* revealing knowledge; the light of knowledge without a shadow; purely illuminating knowledge

SUTRA 2:28

योगाङ्गानुष्ठानादशुद्धिक्षये ज्ञानदीप्तिराविवेकख्यातेः ॥२८॥

yoga-aṅga-anuṣṭhānāt aśuddhi-kṣaye jñāna-dīptiḥ āvivekakhyāteḥ ॥ 28 ॥

The practice of the limbs of yoga destroys impurities; thereafter, knowledge continues to brighten all the way to *viveka khyati*, the domain of unshakeable discernment.

yoga- the practice leading to mastery over the roaming tendencies of the mind; *samādhi*

aṅga- limbs; components; divisions

anuṣṭhānāt *abl. sg. n.* of *anuṣṭhāna*, practice

aśuddhi-kṣaye *loc. sg. m.* of *aśuddhi-kṣaya*, destruction of impurities
aśuddhi, impurity; contamination; *kṣaya*, destruction; deterioration; elimination

jñāna-dīptiḥ *nom. sg. f.* the shine of knowledge; lighting the knowledge

jñāna, knowledge; *dīpti,* shine; illumination; ignition

ā-vivekakhyāteḥ

abl. sg. f. of *āvivekakhyāti,* domain of unshakeable discernment; discerning knowledge that is complete in every sense

ā, from every direction; in every respect; in every sense; *vivekakhyāti,* discerning knowledge

SUTRA 2:29

यमनियमासनप्राणायामप्रत्याहारधारणाध्यान
समाधयोऽष्टावङ्गानि ॥२९॥

yama-niyama-āsana-prāṇāyāma-pratyāhāra-dhāraṇā-dhyāna-samādhayaḥ aṣṭau aṅgāni ॥ 29 ॥

Restraint, observance, physical posture, mastery of the pranic force, recalling the senses, concentration, meditation, and spiritual absorption are the eight components of yoga.

yama- restraint; self-control; withstanding the force of craving

niyama- observance; keeping a firm resolve

āsana- physical posture; steady and comfortable pose

prāṇāyāma- mastery of the pranic force; breathing practice

pratyāhāra- recalling the senses; bringing the forces of the mind and senses to their natural resting place

dhāraṇā-	concentration; retaining the mind; focusing the mind on a chosen object
dhyāna-	meditation; uninterrupted flow of the same or similar cognitions; a prolonged and uninterrupted flow of concentration
samādhayaḥ	*nom. pl. m.* spiritual absorption; perfect stillness; perfectly still, pristine state of mind; a state where the object of cognition, the process of cognition, and the awareness of oneself as a cognizant being have merged in a single, homogeneous awareness
aṣṭau	*nom. pl. n.* eight
aṅgāni	*nom. pl. m.* of *aṅga*, limb; component

SUTRA 2:30

अहिंसासत्यास्तेयब्रह्मचर्यापरिग्रहा यमाः ॥३०॥

ahiṁsā-satya-asteya-brahmacarya-aparigrahāḥ yamāḥ ॥ 30 ॥

Non-violence, truthfulness, non-stealing, continence, and non-possessiveness are the restraints.

ahiṁsā-	non-violence; non-harming; lack of animosity; abiding in the principles of friendliness, love, and compassion
satya-	truthfulness; not lying; constant awareness of the higher reality
asteya-	non-stealing; refraining from having that which is not rightfully ours

brahmacarya-	continence; self-control; conserving sexual energy; directing all psycho-energetic resources to the realization of all-pervading consciousness
aparigrahāḥ	*nom. pl. m.* of *aparigraha,* non-possessiveness; not hoarding; not holding on to one's belongings
yamāḥ	*nom. pl. m.* of *yama,* restraint; self-discipline

SUTRA 2:31

जातिदेशकालसमयानवच्छिन्नाः सार्वभौमा महाव्रतम्
॥३१॥

jāti-deśa-kāla-samaya-anavacchinnāḥ sārva-bhaumāḥ mahā-vratam ॥ 31 ॥

[The aforesaid five restraints] are not affected by the factors of class, place, time, and circumstance. They are universally applicable and constitute the great vow.

jāti-	class; group; race; ethnicity; species
deśa-	place; location; country
kāla-	time
samaya-	circumstance
anavacchinnāḥ	*nom. pl. m.* of *anavacchinna,* that which is not affected or confined
sārva-bhaumāḥ	*nom. pl. m.* universal; pertaining to every aspect of ground or vantage point *sārva,* derived from *sarva,* all; *bhauma,* derived from *bhumi,* ground

mahā-vratam *nom. sg. n.* the great vow; the highest observance
mahā, great; *vratam,* vow; observance; guiding principle

SUTRA 2:32

शौचसंतोषतपःस्वाध्यायेश्वरप्रणिधानानि नियमाः ॥३२॥

śauca-santoṣa-tapaḥ-svādhyāya-īśvara-praṇidhānāni niyamāḥ ॥ 32 ॥

Purity, contentment, austerity, self-study, and trustful surrender to Ishvara are the observances.

śauca- purity; cleanliness; the condition in which light shines

santoṣa- contentment; satisfaction; lack of wanting

tapaḥ- austerity; penance; standing against sense cravings

svādhyāya- self-study; self-reflection; study of scriptures

īśvara-praṇidhānāni
nom. pl. n. trustful surrender to the highest divinity
īśvara, the highest divinity; primordial master, protector, and guide; *praṇidhānāni,* plural of *praṇidhāna,* complete surrender; offering one's actions and the fruits of actions to the divine being

niyamāḥ *nom. pl. m.* of *niyama*, observance; discipline not to be ignored

SUTRA 2:33

वितर्कबाधने प्रतिपक्षभावनम् ॥३३॥

vitarka-bādhane pratipakṣa-bhāvanam ॥ 33 ॥

To arrest afflicting thoughts, cultivate thoughts opposed to them.

vitarka-bādhane
loc. sg. m. of *vitarka-bādhana,* arrest afflicting thoughts; block thoughts full of conflict
vitarka, afflicting thoughts; thoughts full of doubt and contradictions; disturbing thoughts; painful thoughts and feelings;
bādhana, arresting; checking; blocking

pratipakṣa- opposite; counteracting; belonging to the other side

bhāvanam *nom. sg. n.* thinking; contemplating; act of willful thinking

SUTRA 2:34

वितर्का हिंसादयः कृतकारितानुमोदिता
लोभक्रोधमोहपूर्वका मृदुमध्याधिमात्रा
दुःखाज्ञानानन्तफला इति प्रतिपक्षभावनम् ॥३४॥

vitarkāḥ hiṁsādayaḥ kṛta-kārita-anumoditāḥ lobha-krodha-moha-pūrvakāḥ mṛdu-madhya-adhimātrāḥ duḥkha-ajñānā-ananta-phalāḥ iti pratipakṣa-bhāvanam ॥ 34 ॥

Violence and the others are afflicting thoughts. We put these thoughts into action by ourselves, through others, or by tacit consent. These thoughts are propelled by greed, anger, or

confusion. They are mild, intermediate, or intense. We nullify these afflicting thoughts by realizing they bear unending fruit of pain and ignorance.

vitarkāḥ	*nom. pl. m.* of *vitarka*, afflicting thoughts; thoughts full of doubt and contradictions; disturbing thoughts; painful thoughts and feelings
hiṁsā-ādayaḥ	*nom. pl. m.* of *hiṁsā-ādi,* violence, etc. *hiṁsā,* violence; *ādi,* etc.; beginning with; first
kṛta-	done
kārita-	made to do
anumoditāḥ	*nom. pl. m.* consented
lobha-	greed
krodha-	anger
moha-	confusion; delusion
pūrvakāḥ	*nom. pl. m.* preceded by
mṛdu-	mild; gentle
madhya-	intermediate
adhimātrāḥ	*nom. pl. m.* exceedingly intense
duḥkha-	pain
ajñānā-	ignorance; misunderstanding; *avidyā*
ananta-	endless
phalāḥ	*nom. pl. m.* fruits; results
iti	thus

pratipakṣa-	opposite; counteracting; belonging to the other side
bhāvanam	*nom. sg. n.* thinking; contemplating; act of willful thinking

SUTRA 2:35

अहिंसाप्रतिष्ठायां तत्सन्निधौ वैरत्यागः ॥३५॥

ahiṁsā-pratiṣṭhāyāṁ tat-sannidhau vaira-tyāgaḥ ॥ 35 ॥

In the company of a yogi established in non-violence, animosity vanishes.

ahiṁsā-	non-violence
pratiṣṭhāyāṁ	*loc. sg. f.* upon being established
tat-	that
sannidhau	*loc. sg. m.* of *sam-nidhi*, the presence of
vaira-	animosity
tyāgaḥ	*nom. sg. m.* renunciation; absence

SUTRA 2:36

सत्यप्रतिष्ठायां क्रियाफलाश्रयत्वम् ॥३६॥

satya-pratiṣṭhāyāṁ kriyā-phala-āśrayatvam ॥ 36 ॥

When a yogi is established in truthfulness, actions begin to bear fruit.

satya-	truth
pratiṣṭhāyāṁ	*loc. sg. f.* upon being established

kriyā-phala-āśrayatvam

nom. sg. n. the ground for the fructification of the action

kriyā, action; *phala,* fruit; *āśrayatvam,* the essence of the ground

SUTRA 2:37

अस्तेयप्रतिष्ठायां सर्वरत्नोपस्थानम् ॥३७॥

asteya-pratiṣṭhāyāṁ sarva-ratna-upasthānam ॥ 37 ॥

When a yogi is established in non-stealing, all gems manifest.

asteya-	non-stealing
pratiṣṭhāyāṁ	*loc. sg. f.* upon being established
sarva-	all
ratna-	gems
upasthānam	*nom. sg. n.* coming closer; manifestation

SUTRA 2:38

ब्रह्मचर्यप्रतिष्ठायां वीर्यलाभः ॥३८॥

brahmacarya-pratiṣṭhāyāṁ vīrya-lābhaḥ ॥ 38 ॥

A yogi established in continence gains *virya*, the capacity to transmit knowledge.

brahmacarya-	continence; celibacy
pratiṣṭhāyāṁ	*loc. sg. f.* upon being established
vīrya-	vigor; vitality; indomitable shakti
lābhaḥ	*nom. sg. m.* attainment

SUTRA 2:39

अपरिग्रहस्थैर्ये जन्मकथंतासम्बोधः ।।३९।।

aparigraha-sthairye janma-kathantā-sambodhaḥ ॥ 39 ॥

With firmness in non-possessiveness comes complete understanding of the "why-ness" of birth.

aparigraha-	non-possessiveness
sthairye	*loc. sg. m.* of *sthairya,* firmness; steadiness
janma-	birth
kathantā-	essence of "why"
sambodhaḥ	*nom. sg. m.* complete understanding

SUTRA 2:40

शौचात् स्वाङ्गजुगुप्सा परैरसंसर्गः ।।४०।।

śaucāt sva-aṅga-jugupsā paraiḥ asaṁsargaḥ ॥ 40 ॥

From purity arises sensitivity to the unclean nature of one's own body; [that leads to] unmixing with others.

śaucāt	*abl. sg. m.* of *śauca,* purity; the practice of purity
sva-	one's own
aṅga-	limbs and organs
jugupsā	*nom. sg. f.* feeling of impurity
paraiḥ	*ins. pl. m.* toward others
asaṁsargaḥ	*nom. sg. m.* unmixing; non-attachment

SUTRA 2:41

सत्त्वशुद्धिसौमनस्यैकाग्र्येन्द्रियजयात्मदर्शनयोग्यत्वानि च ॥४१॥

sattva-śuddhi-saumanasya-ekāgrya-indriya-jaya-ātma-darśana-yogyatvāni ca ॥ 41 ॥

[From purity arises] the purity of our essential being, a positive mind, one-pointedness, victory over the senses, and the qualification for having direct experience of our self.

sattva-	illuminative property of *buddhi*, the inner intelligence; pure being
śuddhi-	purification
saumanasya-	the essential property of a good mind; a positive mind
ekāgrya-	one-pointed mind
indriya-jaya-	victory over the senses
ātma-	one's self
darśana-	direct experience
yogyatvāni	*nom. pl. n.* deservingness
ca	and

SUTRA 2:42

संतोषादनुत्तमः सुखलाभः ।।४२।।

santoṣāt anuttamaḥ sukha-lābhaḥ ॥ 42 ॥

From contentment comes happiness without equal.

santoṣāt	*abl. sg. m.* of *santoṣa,* contentment
anuttamaḥ	*nom. sg. m.* unsurpassed
sukha-	happiness
lābhaḥ	*nom. sg. m.* attainment

SUTRA 2:43

कायेन्द्रियसिद्धिरशुद्धिक्षयात् तपसः ।।४३।।

kāya-indriya-siddhiḥ aśuddhi-kṣayāt tapasaḥ ॥ 43 ॥

Austerity destroys impurities. From that come yogic accomplishments pertaining to the body and senses.

kāya-	body
indriya-	senses
siddhiḥ	*nom. sg. f.* yogic accomplishment
aśuddhi-	impurity
kṣayāt	*abl. sg. m.* of *kṣaya,* destruction
tapasaḥ	*abl. sg. n.* of *tapaḥ,* austerity

SUTRA 2:44

स्वाध्यायादिष्टदेवतासम्प्रयोगः ॥४४॥

svādhyāyāt iṣṭa-devatā-samprayogaḥ ॥ 44 ॥

From self-study comes the opportunity to be in the company of bright beings [of our choice].

svādhyāyāt	*abl. sg. m.* of *svādhyāya,* self-study
iṣṭa-	desirable; capable of guiding and enlightening
devatā-	intrinsic power of *deva,* the bright being
samprayogaḥ	*nom. sg. m.* union; interaction with

SUTRA 2:45

समाधिसिद्धिरीश्वरप्रणिधानात् ॥४५॥

samādhi-siddhiḥ īśvara-praṇidhānāt ॥ 45 ॥

From trustful surrender to Ishvara comes samadhi.

samādhi-	state of mind beyond all cognitions
siddhiḥ	*nom. sg. f.* yogic accomplishment
īśvara-	all-pervading divine being beyond time and space and absolutely untouched by afflictions
praṇidhānāt	*abl. sg. n.* from trustful surrender

SUTRA 2:46

स्थिरसुखम् आसनम् ॥४६॥

sthira-sukham āsanam ॥ 46 ॥

A stable and comfortable posture is *asana*.

sthira- stable; lasting; unmoving; steady

sukham *nom. sg. n.* comfortable; pleasant

āsanam *nom. sg. n.* posture; seat

SUTRA 2:47

प्रयत्नशैथिल्यानन्तसमापत्तिभ्याम् ॥४७॥

prayatna-śaithilya-ananta-samāpattibhyām ॥ 47 ॥

[Perfection in asana is attained] by loosening of [tension caused by] effort and by [mental] absorption in the infinite.

pra-yatna- special effort

pra, special; precise; superior; *yatna,* effort

śaithilya- derived from *śithila,* loose; relaxed; not tense; *śaithilya* is a state of being relaxed, a stress-free state

ananta- without an end; limitless; infinite; the primordial snake, *śeṣa nāga*; another name for the sage Patanjali

samāpattibhyām

ins. du. m. of *samāpatti,* mental absorption

SUTRA 2:48

ततो द्वन्द्वानभिघातः ॥४८॥

tataḥ dvandva-an-abhi-ghātaḥ ॥ 48 ॥

From that [comes] lack of injury caused by the pairs of opposites.

tataḥ	*abl. sg. n.* from that	
dvandva-	pair; dual; pair of opposites	
an-abhi-ghātaḥ	*nom. sg. m.* lack of injury	*an,* not; lack of; no more; *abhi,* from all around; from every direction; in every respect; *ghāta,* injury

SUTRA 2:49

तस्मिन्सति श्वासप्रश्वासयोर्गतिविच्छेदः प्राणायामः ॥४९॥

tasmin sati śvāsa-praśvāsayoḥ gati-vicchedaḥ prāṇāyāmaḥ ॥ 49 ॥

Complete mastery over the roaming tendencies of inhalation and exhalation is *pranayama*; it is to be practiced only after mastering asana.

tasmin	*loc. sg. n.* after that; upon that
sati	*loc. sg. n.* only then; never without
śvāsa-	inhalation
praśvāsayoḥ	*gen. du. m.* of *praśvāsa*, exhalation
gati-	movement; speed

vicchedaḥ — *nom. sg. m.* cessation; elimination; stopping; controlling

prāṇāyāmaḥ — *nom. sg. m.* composite of *prāṇa* and *āyāma*; expansion of the life force

prāṇa, fundamental principle of pulsation; life force; the force which brings the body of inert matter to life; *āyāma,* composite of the prefix *ā* and *yāma*; *ā,* from every direction; in every respect; in every manner; *yāma,* expansion; stretching

SUTRA 2:50

बाह्याभ्यन्तरस्तम्भवृत्तिर्देशकालसंख्याभिः परिदृष्टो दीर्घसूक्ष्मः ॥५०॥

bāhya-ābhyantara-stambha-vṛttiḥ deśa-kāla-saṁkhyābhiḥ paridṛṣṭaḥ dīrgha-sūkṣmaḥ ॥ 50 ॥

[Pranayama with breath retention could be] threefold: external, internal, or stopping the breath wherever it is. Each is monitored by space, time, and number, and each is characterized by its length and subtlety.

bāhya- — external; outside the body

ābhyantara- — internal; inside the body

stambha- — stopping wherever it is; immobilizing; immobilizing suddenly

vṛttiḥ — *nom. sg. f.* movement; revolving tendency

deśa- — space; place

kāla- — time

saṁkhyābhiḥ	*ins. pl. f.* of *saṁkhyā,* number
paridṛṣṭaḥ	*nom. sg. m.* fully seen; properly monitored; surveyed in every respect and from every direction
dīrgha-	long; prolonged; covering relatively longer time, space, or both
sūkṣmaḥ	*nom. sg. m.* of *sūkṣma,* subtle

SUTRA 2:51

बाह्याभ्यन्तरविषयाक्षेपी चतुर्थः ॥५१॥

bāhya-ābhyantara-viṣaya-ākṣepī caturthaḥ ॥ 51 ॥

The fourth pranayama transcends the domain of external and internal pranayamas.

bāhya-	external
ābhyantara-	internal
viṣaya-	domain; object
ākṣepī	*nom. sg. m.* that which transcends; that which blocks; that which objects
caturthaḥ	*nom. sg. m.* fourth

SUTRA 2:52

ततः क्षीयते प्रकाशावरणम् ॥५२॥

tataḥ kṣīyate prakāśa-āvaraṇam ॥ 52 ॥

The veil over the light is attenuated.

tataḥ	*ab. sg. n.* then
kṣīyate	*3rd person sg.* of the verb *kṣī,* attenuates; weakens; deteriorates
prakāśa-	light; illumination
āvaraṇam	*nom. sg. n.* veil

SUTRA 2:53

धारणासु च योग्यता मनसः ॥५३॥

dhāraṇāsu ca yogyatā manasaḥ ॥ 53 ॥

The mind is also qualified for concentrations.

dhāraṇāsu	*loc. pl. f.* of *dhāraṇā,* concentration
ca	also; and; in addition to
yogyatā	*nom. sg. f.* qualification
manasaḥ	*gen. sg. n.* of *manas,* mind

SUTRA 2:54

स्वविषयासम्प्रयोगे चित्तस्यस्वरूपानुकार इवेन्द्रियाणां प्रत्याहारः ॥५४॥

sva-viṣaya-asamprayoge cittasya svarūpa-anukāraḥ iva indriyāṇāṁ pratyāhāraḥ ॥ 54 ॥

Lacking contact with their respective objects, when senses assume the nature of mind it is *pratyahara*.

sva-	one's own
viṣaya-	object
asamprayoge	*loc. sg. m.* of *asmaprayoga,* lack of contact; lack of union
cittasya	*gen. sg. n.* of mind
svarūpa-	essential nature
anukāraḥ	*nom. sg. m.* appearance
iva	like
indriyāṇāṁ	*gen. pl. m.* of the senses
pratyāhāraḥ	*nom. sg. m.* withdrawing from every direction toward a focal point

SUTRA 2:55

ततः परमा वश्यतेन्द्रियाणाम् ॥५५॥

tataḥ paramā vaśyatā indriyāṇām ॥ 55 ॥

From that [pratyahara] comes the highest level of mastery over the senses.

tataḥ	*abl. sg. n.*	from that
paramā	*nom. sg. f.*	the highest
vaśyatā	*nom. sg. f.*	mastery; victory; control; authority
indriyāṇām	*gen. pl. m.*	of the senses

APPENDIX C

Shat Karma: Six Cleansing Techniques

A clear, steady mind requires a healthy body. A healthy body, in turn, requires a clean, well-balanced internal ecology. Our internal ecology is disturbed by even a minute accumulation of toxins—they disrupt the natural rhythm and secretions of our organs and interfere with healthy absorption. Lack of sensitivity to our internal states, coupled with a lack of connection to our inner intelligence, prevents us from detecting this upheaval in the early stages. We notice it and become alarmed only when our internal ecology has deteriorated to such an extent that our organs have difficulty functioning. We then expend so much energy attending to our health that we have little left for attending to the needs of our mind and soul.

To prevent the accumulation of toxins, yogis recommend *shat karma,* six cleansing techniques that can be adopted as part of a yogic lifestyle. They are *dhauti, basti, neti, trataka, nauli,* and *kapalabhati.*

Dhauti

Dhauti means "washing the upper gastrointestinal tract." In the yoga community it is commonly known as "the upper wash." There are two main techniques: *vastra dhauti* and *jala dhauti*. To do vastra dhauti, slowly swallow a clean, wet cotton cloth, approximately three feet long and three inches wide, and immediately draw it back out of your stomach. To do jala dhauti, drink a liter or more of water on an empty stomach and immediately regurgitate it by stimulating your gag reflex.

Both techniques clean the stomach by removing excess mucus. Dhauti helps with asthma, bronchial disorders, and other respiratory ailments, as well as with disorders of the upper digestive tract. This practice also has a positive effect on eating disorders and on emotional disturbances.

Basti

Basti, a technique for cleaning the colon, involves drawing clean water into the rectum and up into the colon. This is done by inserting a tube into the anus, squatting navel-deep in water, and sucking clean water into the rectum by contracting the anus internally. Those who have not practiced *ashvini mudra* and *uddiyana bandha* will not be able to create a vacuum in the colon and abdominal cavity, and so may be unable to pull the water through the rectum. An enema is a much easier and more accessible way to cleanse the colon.

Basti relieves congestion in the colon and cleans the lower portion of the digestive tract. It alleviates digestive disorders, constipation, sluggish digestion, and general dullness. However, excessive use of basti may damage the mucus membranes lining the colon. Instead, the yogis advise activating and energizing the entire colon with the practice of yogic techniques such as ashvini mudra and *agni sara*. Then, to cleanse the colon, they further advise undertaking *gaja karani,* the complete wash, once or twice a year. This practice, which subsumes both dhauti and basti, cleans the entire gastrointestinal tract.

To do gaja karani, the complete wash, drink a large amount of warm saline water in a relatively short period of time, then squat and stretch gently and repetitively to move the water through the intestinal tract. Continue drinking, stretching, squatting, and defecating until the discharge runs clear. Then drink a large amount of diluted citrus juice for nourishment and to remove excess salt from your body.

The complete wash requires preparation. Just as you must cleanse your intestinal tract the day before a colonoscopy, you must prepare for the complete wash by eating lightly the day before—preferably by taking only vegetable broth, juices, and other liquids. Begin drinking the warm salt water the next morning after you have had your regular bowel movement.

Neti

Neti means "cleansing the nostrils." The primary method is *jala neti,* which involves pouring salt water through one nostril and allowing it to flow through the nose and out the other nostril. The water should be warmer than body temperature but not uncomfortably hot; the salinity should be slightly higher than the normal concentration of salt in the blood.

It is best to learn jala neti from an experienced teacher, but here is a general description of the practice. Use a water pot with a nozzle that fits comfortably in the opening of your nostrils. Position the nozzle in one nostril; bend your head slightly to one side, elevating the pot so that gravity pulls the water into one nostril, through the nose, and out the other nostril. When approximately half of the saline solution is gone, switch nostrils and do the same thing on the other side.

The dual action of salt and warm water dissolves accumulated mucus and washes it away. To remove water trapped in your nasal passage or sinuses, bend forward and blow air through your nose several times.

Trataka

Trataka means "gazing." This practice involves stabilizing the focus of your eyes on a single point until they tear. The object of concentration is usually a candle flame, but tradition may assign a different object.

Trataka accelerates the capacity for concentration while calming brain activity. Stabilizing the gaze brings stability to the mind, because vision is the most active of the senses. Stabilizing the gaze also enables the mind to form the habit of remaining focused on one object, which enhances the ability to arrest the mind's roaming tendencies. The yoga texts also attribute clarity of external vision to this practice.

Nauli

Nauli is an advanced yogic practice that involves churning the abdominal cavity. It is mastered in several steps.

Ashvini mudra is the first step. Gently squeezing and relaxing the anus and the muscles surrounding the rectum enables you to cultivate conscious awareness of this region, an area largely controlled by the autonomic nervous system.

The second step is *mula bandha,* commonly known as "the root lock." Using ashvini mudra as your foundation, simultaneously squeeze and constrict your buttocks, rectum, and perineum, and then lift them up and in toward the interior of the pelvis.

The third step is to use mula bandha as the foundation for *uddiyana bandha,* the navel lock. Uddiyana bandha entails pulling the root lock further up, taking it all the way to the navel center. While exhaling, squeeze your buttocks, rectum, and perineum, and pull them all up toward the pelvis, and then up toward the navel center. This long, deep exhalation creates a vacuum in the pelvic and abdominal cavity. At the peak of the exhalation, pull the entire pelvic and abdominal cavity toward the spine. This is uddiyana bandha. s

Uddiyana bandha is then used as the foundation for *nauli,* churning the abdominal cavity. While retaining uddiyana bandha, isolate the central muscles of the abdomen and, with the power of your intention, use them as a churning rod. Exhale completely and retain the breath, while moving the central abdominal muscles from right to left and left to right in a wavelike motion.

It may take a beginning student 6 to 12 months to master this practice, but the rewards are enormous. Nauli strengthens the lower back, energizes and nourishes all the organs in this area, and eventually engenders voluntary control over involuntary muscles. For ages, nauli has been used to ignite the inner fire and conquer a spiritual aspirant's greatest enemies—sloth and hopelessness.

Kapalabhati

Kapalabhati is one of the breathing techniques designed to activate and energize the brain. Mastery of mula bandha—the ability to maintain root lock effortlessly—is a prerequisite. Without mula bandha there is no kapalabhati, because if mula bandha demands attention it will be impossible to employ the mind to attend the practice of kapalabhati.

To do the practice, sit in a meditative pose with your head, neck, and trunk aligned. In this practice, make your exhalation deep and forceful and your inhalation gentle. Make both exhalation and inhalation rapid. Fully engage your abdominal muscles but have little movement in the chest. Make the movement in the abdominal region vigorous, but do not let your mind be distracted by the movement. Rather, keep your mind free to observe the subtle response to this vigorous breathing deep inside the brain. The brain may be aware of the whole body but it is not aware of itself. The practice of kapalabhati eventually leads to an awareness of the subtle nuances in the brain center—the greatest of all mysteries. This awareness will allow you to energize the brain to more effectively govern and guide the functions of the body.

APPENDIX D

Agni Sara

Agni sara is the most effective practice for reaching the core of our body, shaking off deep-rooted inertia, awakening the gut brain, and providing nourishment to all organ systems. Yogis of the tantric tradition, particularly those belonging to the *samaya* school, claim that, taken together, the fruit of practicing *asanas*, *bandhas*, and *mudras* barely yields one-sixteenth of the fruit of practicing agni sara.

In addition to providing numerous physical, mental, and pranic benefits, agni sara is the gateway to the most advanced practices of yoga and tantra. For example, the practice described in *Yoga Sutra* 3:29 leading to comprehending *kaya vyuha,* the complex formation of the human body, is possible only after gaining proficiency in agni sara. Similarly, the practices of meditating on the sun or on the solar plexus (YS 3:26) and the practice of discovering *kaya sampat*, the extraordinary powers buried in the human body (YS 3:46), require the firm foundation of proficiency in agni sara. Practicing mantras vested with the power to make invisible forces of nature visible can have a catastrophic effect if the extraordinary forces at the *manipura chakra* are not awakened by advanced practices like agni sara. Highly evolved tantric rituals, such as *rudra yaga* and those pertaining to Durga, Tara, Chinnamasta, Bagalamukhi, and Sri Vidya, will have a lasting transformative effect only when an aspirant has gained access to the manipura chakra and has cultivated sensitivity to its intrinsic transformative power. Agni sara is one of the most reliable ways of gaining access to the manipura chakra.

The practices of *nauli* and *kapalabhati* described in Appendix C are subsumed in agni sara. In other words, the practices of *ashvini mudra, mula bandha,* and *uddiyana bandha* are prerequisites for practicing agni sara. The practice itself is best learned directly from an adept. Traditionally, agni sara is taught in seven steps, each of which has prerequisites and precautions.

As a standard rule, practice agni sara only when the colon is clean and the bladder is empty. Do not practice when you are hungry or thirsty.

Before you engage in the practice, do some simple stretches to remove general inertia and stiffness. With the help of postures that involve forward bends, backward bends, and side bends, free your spinal column, especially the lower back, hips, and pelvic and abdominal cavities.

Here is a brief description of the first step of agni sara:

Stand firmly with your feet approximately 12 inches apart. Bend your knees and place your hands on your thighs just above the knees, transferring the weight of your torso onto your thighs, keeping your arms straight.

Bring your attention to the region of the perineum. With a deep, smooth, slow exhalation, begin squeezing your buttocks in and up from all sides—front, back, and both sides. At the peak of the exhalation, give a final push by squeezing your anus muscles as intensely as possible. Then, with the inhalation, let your muscles disengage and return to their normal position. Repeat the practice 10 to 25 times. This practice should give you a sense of relief rather than discomfort. You should feel refreshed and energized. Exhaustion is a sign that you are not doing the practice correctly.

After a few weeks or months, add one more element. Bring your attention to the left side of your groin and transfer some of your weight to the left foot. With the next exhalation, instead of squeezing your buttocks in and up from all directions, begin pulling up the muscles in your left inner thigh and left groin more strongly than the muscles on the right side. To intensify the upward pull, lift your left ankle slightly, transfer the weight of your body to your left big toe, and tilt your left knee inward. Feel as though your exhalation is starting from your toe and is lifting your left leg energetically, while your left big toe remains firmly anchored on the ground. With the combined forces of your breath and intention, continue pulling the energy up through your left foot, inner calf, inner thigh, and groin—all the way to where the left side of your abdominal cavity meets your lower ribs. By the time you reach your ribs, the exhalation is completed and there is no room to pull your energy up further. Now inhale gently—this is a completely passive process. While you are inhaling, the muscles in the left side of your body—from the lower ribs all the way to your toes—return to their normal position.

With the next exhalation, repeat the entire process, this time focusing on the right side. Alternate from side to side for 15 to 20 breaths, but avoid becoming exhausted.

When you have mastered this first step, you will be able to sense the pranic counterpart of your physical frame. This sensitivity will eventually empower you to heal and energize your body, especially the organs in the area of the first three chakras. You will become acutely aware of the pranic flow that supplies energy and intelligence to your muscles and nervous system.

This first step serves as the foundation for all the subsequent steps.

APPENDIX E

Prana Anusandhana

We all breathe, yet few of us know anything about the subtle anatomy of the breath. For most of us, breathing is a physiological process—one that runs on autopilot. We inhale and air goes in; we exhale and air goes out. Science tells us our primitive brain regulates our breathing, but beyond that, what makes us inhale and exhale remains a mystery to us. Yogis call this mystery *prana*. *Prana anusandhana* is a process whereby we become aware of the difference between breathing and what makes us breathe. In the absence of this awareness, the advanced stages of pranayama—including *prana samvedana, prana samrodha,* and the four pranayamas described in the *Yoga Sutra*—remain confined to the domain of physical exercise. They have little or no spiritual value. Traditionally, prana anusandhana is taught in seven steps.

The **first step** is *aharana pranayama. Aharana* means "to bring back." Aharana pranayama involves bringing our prana shakti back to its home base. Our body—more precisely, the heart—is the residence of prana. Mind and prana live together and work together. When the mind is scattered, prana is scattered. Before we can pull our prana back to its main seat in the heart, we have to first become aware of the union of prana and mind. This is a subtle process and should not be mistaken for a breathing exercise.

To practice aharana pranayama, assume your most comfortable sitting posture. Close your eyes and become aware of your body and the space around your body. Bring your attention to your inhalation and exhalation, and make sure there is no shakiness or noise in your breath. With the power of your intention, relax your shoulders. Mentally check the position of your spine—sit straight and avoid creating an exaggerated arch. Breathe without making an effort.

If your mind is not fully engaged in experiencing your body, but is instead chasing the objects of your thoughts, your breath will be choppy and erratic. Due to underdeveloped mental acuity, you may not notice the relationship between a distracted mind and erratic breath, but if you are hooked to a biofeedback machine, you will see it on the screen. If you command your mind to observe the serene flow of your breath, the mind will automatically become quiet, and prana will become quiet in direct proportion to this mental quietude. Experiencing this quietude is becoming aware of the union of prana and mind.

In the same way that effort is detrimental to mastering asana, in the practice of aharana pranayama, making an effort to withdraw the prana and mind from the different quarters of the objective world is a recipe for failure. Pulling the prana and mind back to the center of the heart is an effortless process. Aharana pranayama involves witnessing the smooth flow of the inhalation and exhalation. The resolve to witness the breath automatically withdraws the mind and prana from the outside world. Maintain this awareness for a few minutes before moving on to the next step.

The **second step** is *samikarana pranayama. Samikarana* means "to equalize." Samikarana pranayama involves creating a condition where the quietude of the body is equal to that of the breath. This is accomplished by witnessing the presence of the mind and prana in different parts of the body.

After maintaining aharana pranayama for a few minutes, bring your attention to the crown of your head. Feel the presence of your own being in the region of your fontanel. Do not apply any pressure on your eyes, and do not imagine yourself in a particular form or shape. This is simply a feeling of "presence." Take a few serene breaths and become established in this self-presence. Awareness of your self-presence means you have discovered a point in the space at the crown of your head, and that space is filled with the feeling of I-am-ness. Maintaining this feeling is witnessing, which includes experiencing the unity of prana and mind.

While remaining aware of this particular point in the region of your crown, take a deep breath. Feel as though your head, particularly the region of the fontanel, is filled with breath. Then begin exhaling, letting your mind descend through the front of your body—first to your forehead, then to the center between your eyebrows, nostrils, throat, heart, sternum, navel center, pelvis, and all the way to your perineum. By the time your reach the perineum, your exhalation is completed.

Without pausing, begin inhaling with the awareness of ascending through the back of your body, paying attention to the areas parallel to the pelvis, navel center, sternum, heart, throat, nostrils, eyebrows, and forehead. In other words, while exhaling, descend from the crown to the perineum through the front of your body, and while inhaling, ascend from the perineum to the crown through the back of your body. Including the crown and perineum, there are ten specific spaces in which you are emphasizing the process of witnessing yourself (i.e., your mind and prana). This process fills your body with the quietude inherent in your mind and prana. Repeat this process 10 to 12 times before moving to the next step.

The **third step**, *dirgha-prashvasa pranayama,* requires some effort. In this pranayama, the exhalation is longer than the inhalation *(dirgha-prashvasa* means "long exhalation"). Once again, feel your breath descending from the crown of the head to the perineum with the exhalation, and ascending from the perineum to the crown with the inhalation, but this time do not differentiate between the front and back of the body: let your exhalation and inhalation move downward and upward while sweeping the entire body. Furthermore, while adhering to the principle of effortlessness, exhale as slowly and deeply as possible. This will enable you to lengthen the exhalation. The longer it takes to exhale, the easier it will be to inhale absolutely effortlessly. In other words, make a slight effort to prolong your exhalation, but make no effort to prolong your inhalation.

In attempting to prolong the exhalation, do not push yourself too hard. If you are experiencing an urgent need to inhale by the time your exhalation is about to reach the perineum, you have put too much effort into extending it. This will cause discomfort in the region of your heart, which will create tension in the lungs and diaphragm. You will gasp for air. Rushing to inhale will take away the serene quality of your inhalation. To avoid this, follow the golden rule of asana: *sthiram,* stability, and *sukham,* comfort. Practice steadily at a comfortable pace while applying the principle of effortless effort. Dirgha-prashvasa pranayama engenders a sense of alertness, regulates the functions of the diaphragm, lungs, and heart, and helps to remove toxins from the bloodstream.

The **fourth step** is *nadi shodhana pranayama.* The distinguishing feature of this pranayama is that you inhale through one nostril and exhale from the other. Sit with your head, neck, and trunk comfortably erect. After a deep inhalation, close your right nostril with your right thumb and exhale slowly through the left nostril. At the end of the exhalation, close your left nostril with your ring finger and inhale slowly and deeply through your right nostril. At the end of the inhalation, close your right nostril and exhale through the left. Following this pattern, exhale three times through the left nostril and inhale three times through the right. This completes one cycle. Then take three normal breaths through both nostrils before beginning the second cycle. This time, begin exhaling through the right nostril and inhale through the left. After three exhalations and inhalations, again take three normal breaths.

Nadi shodhana demands more effort than dirgha-prashvasa, and its effect is more precise. It balances mutually supporting forces of the sun and moon, yin and yang, and the masculine and feminine energies. This balancing action is engendered by harmonizing the sympathetic and parasympathetic nervous systems. The end result is the purification of the *nadis,* energy channels, which support and nourish both the body and the mind.

The **fifth step** is *anuloma pranayama. Anuloma* means "to follow the same trail." In this pranayama, you exhale and inhale through the same nostril rapidly and forcefully. A stable and comfortable sitting posture is even more crucial in this step than in the four previous steps. Make sure your spine is straight, your shoulders and abdomen are relaxed, and your waist is not restricted. In this pranayama, as well as in the two that follow, it is necessary to apply mula bandha.

To practice anuloma, inhale deeply, then close the right nostril with the right thumb. Exhale through the left nostril as forcefully as possible and immediately inhale with equal force through the same nostril. Exhale and inhale in this manner 10 to 12 times before completing the cycle with a forceful, deep, and prolonged exhalation. Before beginning the next cycle, take 5 to 10 normal breaths through both nostrils to restore stability and comfort. Then start the second cycle. This time, close your left nostril with your ring finger and exhale and inhale forcefully through the right nostril. After 10 to 12 breaths, end the cycle with a forceful, deep, and prolonged exhalation. Once again take 5 to 10 normal breaths before moving on to the sixth step of the practice.

Anuloma pranayama and the remaining two pranayamas—*viloma* and *pratiloma*—energize the visceral organs, strengthen the nervous system, and ignite the fire at the navel center.

The **sixth step** is *viloma pranayama. Viloma* means "to follow the reverse trail." In this pranayama, you exhale from one nostril and inhale from the other. Both inhalation and exhalation are rapid and forceful. Close your right nostril and exhale through the left. At the end of the exhalation, close the left nostril and inhale forcefully through the right. Take 10 to 12 breaths in this manner, completing the cycle with a forceful exhalation through the left nostril. Take 5 to 10 normal breaths to restore stability and comfort, then switch nostrils.

You can do this practice as rapidly as you wish, provided your fingers are cooperating in switching back and forth from one nostril to the other. Use as much force as you can without harming your nasal passages.

The **final step** is *pratiloma pranayama. Pratiloma* means "to switch the trails back and forth." Do not practice this pranayama until you have mastered anuloma and viloma pranayamas. In this pranayama, exhale and inhale twice through one nostril, then switch to the other nostril, exhale and inhale twice through that nostril, and then switch again. Both exhalation and inhalation are rapid and forceful.

These last three pranayamas—pratiloma in particular—are not meant for those with weak constitutions. However, a student with a weak constitution who practices asana methodically, and who sequentially and systematically follows the first six steps of prana anusandhana, will become strong enough to practice pratiloma pranayama.

APPENDIX F

Pronunciation and Transliteration Guide

Sanskrit letters form an organized arrangement of sounds, beginning with vowels and concluding with consonants. Each letter corresponds to only one sound. The following pronunciations are approximate; it is helpful to listen to a recording of the alphabet for accuracy.

Vowels in Sanskrit are either short or long. In transliteration, a horizontal line placed over the short vowels (a, i, u, and ṛ) indicates lengthening. Diphthongs (e, ai, o, and au) are long and do not require a diacritical mark. When spoken, long vowels and diphthongs sound about twice as long as short vowels.

a	b**u**t
ā	c**o**t
i	p**i**t
ī	k**ee**p
u	s**u**ture
ū	f**oo**d
ṛ	**ri**d

ṝ	**ree**d
e	l**a**te
ai	**ai**sle
o	t**o**te
au	l**ou**d
aṁ	nasalization of the preceding vowel (s**ung**)
aḥ	a slight aspiration of the preceding vowel (**aha**)

Consonants fall into five classes, starting at the back of the throat and working forward to the lips. Each class is, in turn, divided into five categories: unaspirated or aspirated, unvoiced or voiced, and a nasal sound.

1. The guttural consonants are pronounced from the back of the throat:

k	kid
kh	packhorse
g	give
gh	bighorn
ṅ	ring

2. The palatal consonants are pronounced from the soft palate:

c	chip
ch	pinchhit
j	jump
jh	lodgehouse
ñ	piñata

3. The cerebral consonants are pronounced with the tip of the tongue contacting the roof of the mouth (a retroflex placement signified by a dot under the letter):

ṭ	tar
ṭh	can't handle
ḍ	dart
ḍh	landhunter
ṇ	under

4. The dental consonants are pronounced with the tip of tongue behind the upper row of teeth:

t	tell
th	pothandle
d	dot
dh	headhunter
n	nod

5. The labial consonants are pronounced with the lips:

p	putt
ph	mophead
b	but
bh	labhead
m	mop

Semi-vowels narrow the stream of air, creating friction as the air passes through the mouth:

y	yes
r	rapid
l	lap
v	halfway between wa (wow) and va (vow)

Sibilants include two variants of sh. In practice, they sound about the same:

ś	shove
ṣ	shallow
s	sunny
h	hot

Glossary

abhinivesha Fear of death; the fifth and final affliction.

abhyasa Generally translated as "practice." In the *Yoga Sutra*, it is used precisely to mean making an ardent effort to create and maintain an internal environment in which the mind is allowed to flow peacefully inward.

aghora Literally, "not fierce." In the tantric tradition, it refers to the most benevolent, compassionate, and liberating power of the divine being.

agni sara An advanced practice to lift the energies of the first and second chakras and unite them with the energy of the third chakra. Asana, pranayama, bandha, and mudra are subsumed in this practice.

ahimsa The virtue of non-violence.

aishvarya The intrinsic power of Ishvara.

aparigraha The virtue of non-possessiveness.

apavarga Ultimate freedom; the highest goal of life.

asamprajnata samadhi The highest state of samadhi; samadhi without cognition; the state of perfect spiritual absorption.

asana Posture; a pose characterized by stability and comfort; one of the eight limbs of yoga.

ashakti A state of disempowerment.

ashtanga yoga Eight limbs of yoga, collectively known as *raja yoga* or *Patanjala Yoga*.

asmita The sense of I-am-ness; the second of the five afflictions.
asteya The virtue of non-stealing.
avidya Ignorance; the first of the five afflictions and the mother of all afflictions.
bhautika sarga The manifestation of the universe pertaining to the physical world.
bhoga Fulfillment; one of the two fundamental goals of life.
bindu Point of reference; in tantra and kundalini yoga, it refers to the concentrated field of energy at different chakras, particularly at the navel and in the center of the forehead.
brahmacharya Continence; the practice designed to preserve and nurture life-sustaining energy.
buddhi sattva The essence of pure intelligence.
chakra Wheel of energy; center of consciousness.
chaturtha pranayama Literally, the "fourth pranayama"; breathing practice characterized by sensing the subtle flow of prana.
chiti shakti The power of consciousness; self-luminous being; our essential self.
chitta The vast storehouse of samskaras; a term that encompasses all mental faculties; the mind.
chitta vimukti Freedom from the mind and its contents.
devata The essence of the shining being; self-effulgence; deity.
dharana Concentration; one of the eight limbs of yoga.
dharma megha samadhi Literally, "the samadhi of the cloud of dharma"; the transitional state between lower and higher samadhi.
dhyana Meditation; one of the eight limbs of yoga.
dvesha Compelling dislike; the fourth of the five afflictions.
ghora Literally, "fierce." In tantric literature, it refers to the divine emanation frightening to those who are ignorant.
ghora-ghora-tara Literally, "fiercer than the most fierce." In tantric literature, it refers to the divine emanation that has no tolerance for ignorance.
hatha yoga The practices of yoga designed to harmonize the solar and lunar, masculine and feminine, and active and passive forces in our body and mind.

iccha shakti The power of will and determination; in the tantric tradition of Sri Vidya, it is represented by the goddess Kameshvari.
ishta devata The essence of the divine being most compatible with our taste and liking; our chosen deity.
Ishvara pranidhana Trustful surrender to the divine being.
japa Remembering a mantra with feeling.
jiva The individual self.
jnana shakti The power of knowledge; in the tantric tradition of Sri Vidya, it is represented by the goddess Vajreshvari.
kaivalya The state of absoluteness; the highest goal of yoga.
kapha Literally, "phlegm"; the grounding property of nature.
karma Fruit of action; end result.
karmashaya The repository of karma; the mind field where samskaras are stored; the mind.
karya vimukti Freedom from action and its result.
kaya kalpa Rejuvenation of the body; complete healing.
klesha Affliction; the fundamental source of suffering. Affliction is fivefold: *avidya* (ignorance), *asmita* (sense of I-am-ness), *raga* (attachment), *dvesha* (aversion), and *abhinivesha* (fear of death).
kriya Action.
kriya shakti The power of action; in the tantric tradition of Sri Vidya, it is represented by the goddess Bhagamalini.
kriya yoga Yoga in action; a technical term for *tapas, svadhyaya,* and *Ishvara pranidhana.*
kumbhaka Breath retention.
kundalini shakti The dormant force of intelligence.
mahat Literally, "great"; the first evolute of prakriti; the evolutionary state composed of total intelligence.
mahat tattva Same as mahat.
marma-sthana Vital point in the human body.
niyama Literally, "restraint"; one of the eight limbs of yoga.
pitta Literally, "bile"; the fiery property of nature.
prajna Intuition; the field of intuitive wisdom.
prakriti The primordial cause of the universe; the intrinsic power of pure consciousness.

prakritilaya Dissolved in prakriti; a special category of yogi who dies while established in *asmita anugata samadhi* and thus reincarnates with his wisdom and experience intact.

prana Life force.

prana shakti The same as prana.

pranayama Expansion of prana; mastery over *prana shakti*; yogic breathing techniques.

pratipaksha bhavana Contemplating on thoughts contrary to negative thoughts.

pratyahara Withdrawing the mind from the sensory realm and restraining it in an assigned space.

pratyaya sarga The world of mental cognition; the manifestation of our mental world.

purusha Pure consciousness.

raga Attachment; the third of the five afflictions.

raja yoga The tradition of yoga characterized by its eight limbs, as described in the *Yoga Sutra.*

rajas One of the three intrinsic attributes of primordial nature; the principle of pulsation.

samadhi A perfectly still, pristine state of mind; a state of mind free from all karmic impressions.

samprajnata samadhi Lower samadhi; samadhi with cognition.

santosha Contentment.

satkaryavada The doctrine of Sankhya Yoga that holds that the effect exists in the cause.

sattva One of the three intrinsic attributes of primordial nature; the principle of illumination.

satya The virtue of truthfulness.

shakti matra Sheer power; the highest degree of karmic purity, in which karmic impressions are transformed into the pure energy of prakriti.

shakti sadhana Yoga practice which emphasizes the awakening of kundalini shakti.

shastra Texts documenting valid experiences.

shaucha The virtue of purity.

siddha An accomplished master.

Sri Vidya The most exalted tantric tradition, which views the highest being as mother.

svabhava One's own intrinsic attribute; intrinsic nature; the essential characteristic that defines our being.

svadhyaya Self-study; the study of scriptures documenting valid experiences.

tamas One of the three intrinsic attributes of primordial nature; the principle of inertia and darkness.

tanmatra Literally, "that alone"; the subtlest state of evolution, which contains the potential for the world made of matter and energy.

tapas Austerity; heat; a discipline or observance to cleanse the body and purify the mind; a spiritual practice to transcend our physical and mental limitations.

tattva Literally, "the essence of that"; a term signifying evolutionary stages.

Tripura Literally, "three cities"; a term synonymous with Sri Vidya.

vairagya Loosely translated as "non-attachment"; literally, "non-coloring, non-smearing." Vairagya refers to the process of detaching ourselves from our karmic impressions.

vata Literally, "air"; the pulsating property of nature.

videha Beyond body or transcendence of body; a special category of yogi who dies firmly established in the experience of self-luminous joy and thus reincarnates with his knowledge and experience intact.

vritti Thought construct; modification of the mind; a mental cognition that settles in the mind as an impression and later compels us to perform similar actions.

yama Literally, "controller"; one of the eight limbs of yoga.

Index of Citations

Subject Index

anugraha (divine grace), 38, 40
anuloma pranayama, 357–358
aparigraha (non-possessiveness), 164, 167–168, 181, 194–196
apavarga (freedom), 37, 98–100, 125, 127, 128–130
arjana tushti, 142–143
asamprajnata samadhi, 19, 64, 152–153
asana (posture), xii, xiii, 223–239
    agni sara as culmination of, 192–193, 200, 238–239, 349–352
    ananta samapatti, 231, 234–235
    avoiding injury and maintaining health through, 236–239
    criteria for perfection in, 231–235
    defined, 223–226
    effortlessness and lack of tension in, 231–235
    five afflictions, overcoming, 31
    as foundation for other practices, 224–225
    kaya kalpa and, 210
    kaya sampat, discovering, 226–230
    objective world and, 225–226
    pranayama only to be practiced after mastery of, 241, 242
    precision, importance of, 231
    sequencing movements and increasing intensity, 237–238
    stability and comfort in, 223–230
    threshold of discomfort, working up to, 233
ashakti (disempowerment), 33, 37, 106, 112, 139–145, 183
ashtanga yoga, 224, 225. *See also* eight limbs of yoga
ashvini mudra, 344, 347, 350
asmita (I-am-ness or false sense of self-identity), x, 43–47
    abhinivesha and, 54–55, 56
    avidya as basis for, 23, 26–27, 43, 44, 45, 48, 57, 77, 138
    buddhi, as extension of, 125
    consciousness and, 44–46, 48
    defined, 43–44
    dvesha and, 52
    individual soul as, 118–119
    possessiveness rooted in, 184
    raga and, 48–49
asteya (non-stealing), 164, 167–168, 181, 189–190
atman, 27, 280
atripti tushti, 142–143
attachment. *See* raga
attenuated state. *See* tanu
atulya jatiya, 101, 107
austerity. *See* tapas
avairagya, 126
avastha (condition), 115
aversion. *See* dvesha
avidya (ignorance), x, 36–42
    benevolent dimension of, 39–42
    consciousness and, 93
    defined, 22–23, 36–37
    eight limbs of yoga attenuating, 161–162
    Ishvara pranidhana and, 15
    prakriti and our coming into being, 37–41
    as root of all other afflictions, 23, 26–27, 77, 93, 138
    samadhi, as obstacle to, 21
    samsara and, 55
    self-defense, urge for, 165–166
    sva buddhi ("our" mind) deriving from, 137–145
    as veil over our luminosity, 260–261
    vidya and, 36, 37, 41–42, 81
    viparyaya jnana vasana as, 162
    viveka khyati and disappearance of, 159
avishesha, 114, 115–119, 120
ayu, 74, 84, 108

remaining eight limbs of yoga and, 222
sattva, alignment with, 99
svadhyaya leading to, 218, 222
tapas and, 222

jala dhauti, 344
jala neti, 345–346
japa, 9–11, 213, 216–217, 219
jatavedas, 120
jati, 74, 84, 108
Jesus, 185, 187
jiva, 123
jiva bhava, 46. *See also* asmita
jivan-mukta, 63–64, 101, 127, 151
jnana shakti, 4, 96, 126
jnana vritti, 33, 73
jnana yoga, 224
joy. *See* ananda
jyotishmati, 5, 103

Kaitabha, 105
kaivalya, 33, 63, 148, 150
kala tushti, 142
Kali, 105, 250
kapalabhati, 348, 350
kapha, 207–209
Kapila, 37, 38, 111
Karkotaka, 105
karma, 68–89
categories of, 70, 75–76
defined, 3
five afflictions and, 68–70, 73–75
inexorability of, 178
modifying, 75–76, 86
pleasure and pain accompanying, 77–79
samsara and, 74–75
karma bhumi, 126
karma samskara chakra, 82–83, 172
karma vipaka (karmic fruition), 25, 55, 71–76, 94, 108
karma yoga, 3, 224
karya vimukti, 154–156, 159
kaya kalpa (bodily rejuvenation), 17, 209–211
kaya sampat (intrinsic bodily wealth), 211, 226, 349
kaya siddhi (bodily perfection), 5, 206, 211
kevali, 63, 102, 157
kleshas. *See* five afflictions
kliva (powerlessness), 58
knowledge
ignorance (*See* avidya)
power of (jnana shakti), 4, 96, 126
prajna (intuitive wisdom), 153–158, 187
prajna shakti, 170
vidya (knowledge), 36, 37, 41–42, 81
kripana (inability to let go), 58
kriya shakti (power of action), 3–4, 96
kriya yoga
defined, xiii, 3–5
goals of, 249
Ishvara pranidhana and, 5, 11–16, 17, 160, 213 (*See also* Ishvara pranidhana)
meditation and, 66–67
prakriti and, 1, 2–3
samadhi as goal of, 1–2, 18–21, 161
svadhyaya and, 5, 8–11, 16, 17, 160, 213 (*See also* svadhyaya)
tapas and, 5–8, 16–17, 160, 213 (*See also* tapas)
kshaya tushti, 142–143
kumbhaka (breath retention), 245–249
kundalini shakti, 209–210, 234, 241, 249, 253
kundalini yoga, 191, 223, 225, 249

samadhi siddhi, 222
samaya school, 349
samikarana pranayama, 355–356
samprajnata samadhi, 152
samsara (cycle of birth and death)
  aparigraha and, 195
  avidya and, 55
  breaking out of, 61
  grace, escape from cycle as, 222
  gunas and, 83–85
  jaṭi, ayu, and bhoga, 74, 84, 108
  karma and, 74–75
  maha pretas and, 221
  memories of, 53–54
  purpose of, 38–40, 53, 54
samskaras. *See also* five afflictions
  difficulty of putting aside, 15–16
  gunas contaminated by, 106–107
  mind absorbing, 93–94
  power of seeing hindered by, 121–124
  pratyahara and, 270–271, 275
  self-created objective world constructed from, 97
  strengthening with age, 82
samyag-darshana, 87
samyag-drishti, 85
Sanaka, 103
Sanandana, 103
Sanatkumara, 103
Sanatsujata, 103
sankalpa siddhi (perfection of will), 211, 212
Sankhya Yoga
  five afflictions and, 37, 39, 43
  on objective world, 95, 106, 111, 113, 114, 118
  on pain and suffering, 90–92
santosha (contentment), 171, 172, 181–182, 202–203
Sarasvati, 105, 250
sarva-bhava-adhishthatritva, 34
sarvajnatva, 34
satisfactions. *See* tushtis
satkaryavada, 39, 95, 98, 112
sattamatra, 116
sattva. *See* gunas
sattvic tapas, 206
satya (truthfulness), 164, 167–168, 181, 186–188
scriptures. *See also specific texts, and* **Index of Citations**
  shastra kripa (grace of scripture), 11
  study of, 10–11
seeing, power of, 121–124, 131, 146–148, 157, 221
seer and seen, union of, 90–94, 110, 127, 131, 146, 157, 221
seers. *See* rishis
self-defense, urge for, 165–166
self-identity, false sense of. *See* asmita
self-study or self-reflection. *See* svadhyaya
self-trust, lack of. *See* nirahankara
senses
  of action and cognition, 114–115, 139
  ekadasha-indriya-vadha (injury of the eleven senses), 139–140
  indriya siddhi (perfection of the senses), 5, 206–207, 211–212
  withdrawing (*See* pratyahara)
sensuality. *See* abrahmacharya
serpents. *See* snakes and serpents
seven sages, 103
sexual continence. *See* brahmacharya
shabda, 143–144
shakti. *See* power
shakti matra (sheer power), 33, 55, 73
shakti sadhana, kriya yoga as, 5
shaktipata (transmission of spiritual energy), 191, 193
shambhavi mudra, 192
Shankaracharya, 133
shastra kripa (grace of scripture), 11

About the Author

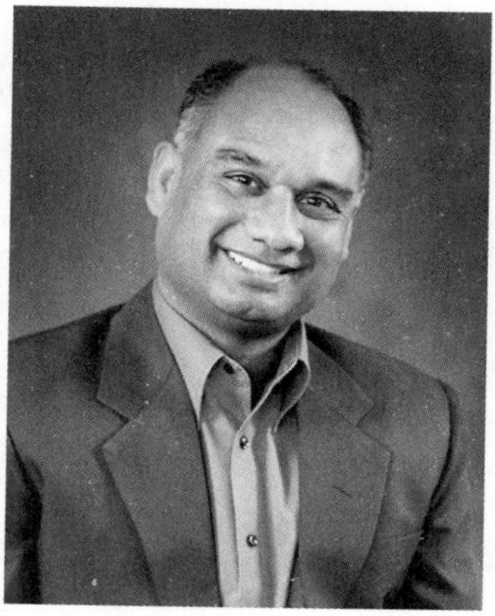

Spiritual head and chairman of the Himalayan Institute, Pandit Rajmani Tigunait, PhD, is the successor of Swami Rama of the Himalayas. Lecturing and teaching worldwide for nearly 40 years, he is the author of 18 books, including his latest, *Sri Sukta: Tantra of Inner Prosperity*, as well as groundbreaking commentaries on the *Yoga Sutra* of Patanjali—*The Secret of the Yoga Sutra: Samadhi Pada* and *The Practice of the Yoga Sutra: Sadhana Pada*. He is a regular contributor to the Himalayan Institute's online Wisdom Library, the driving force of the Institute's global humanitarian projects, and the visionary behind the Institute's consecrated Sri Vidya Shrine in Honesdale, Pennsylvania.

Pandit Tigunait holds two doctorates: one in Sanskrit from the University of Allahabad in India, and another in Oriental studies from the University of Pennsylvania. Family tradition gave Pandit Tigunait access to a vast range of spiritual wisdom preserved in both the written and oral traditions. Before meeting his master, Pandit Tigunait studied Sanskrit, the language of the ancient scriptures of India, as well as the languages of the Buddhist, Jaina, and Zoroastrian traditions. In 1976, Swami Rama ordained Pandit Tigunait into the 5,000-year-old lineage of the Himalayan Masters.

HIMALAYAN INSTITUTE®

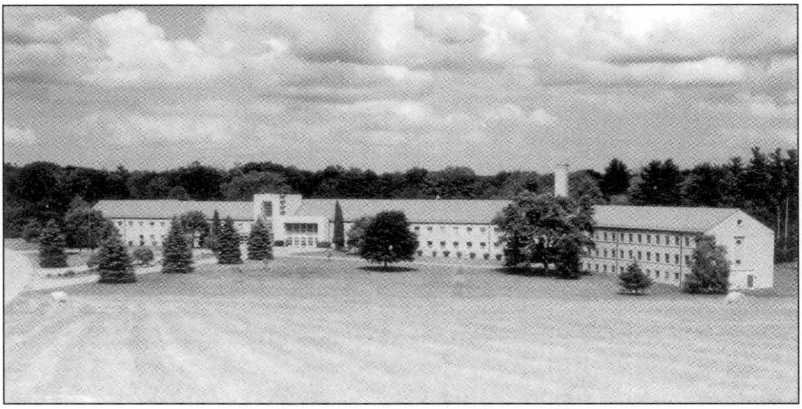

The main building of the Himalayan Institute headquarters near Honesdale, Pennsylvania

The Himalayan Institute

A leader in the field of yoga, meditation, spirituality, and holistic health, the Himalayan Institute is a nonprofit international organization dedicated to serving humanity through educational, spiritual, and humanitarian programs. The mission of the Himalayan Institute is to inspire, educate, and empower all those who seek to experience their full potential.

Founded in 1971 by Swami Rama of the Himalayas, the Himalayan Institute and its varied activities and programs exemplify the spiritual heritage of mankind that unites East and West, spirituality and science, ancient wisdom and modern technology.

Our international headquarters is located on a beautiful 400-acre campus in the rolling hills of the Pocono Mountains of northeastern Pennsylvania. Our spiritually vibrant community and peaceful setting provide the perfect atmosphere for seminars and retreats, residential programs, and holistic health services. Students from all over the world join us to attend diverse programs on subjects such as hatha yoga, meditation, stress reduction, ayurveda, and yoga and tantra philosophy.

In addition, the Himalayan Institute draws on roots in the yoga tradition to serve our members and community through the following programs, services, and products.

Mission Programs

The essence of the Himalayan Institute's teaching mission flows from the timeless message of the Himalayan Masters, including its founder, Swami Rama, and is echoed in our on-site and online mission programming: first we need to become aware of the reality within ourselves, and then we need to build a bridge between our inner and outer worlds. We seek to bring you the best of an authentic tradition, distilled for the modern seeker.

Our mission programs express a rich body of experiential wisdom, focused on yoga and meditation practice and philosophy, including our flagship Vishoka Meditation offerings. In-person mission programs are offered year-round at our campus in Honesdale, Pennsylvania, and include seminars, retreats, and teacher training certification programs.

The Institute is also a leader in hybrid in-person/online education. It offers a wide range of live online courses and certification programs, as well as on-demand digital courses. Join us in person or online to find wisdom from the heart of the yoga tradition, guidance for authentic practice, and a vibrant global community of like-minded seekers.

Wisdom Library and Mission Membership

The Himalayan Institute's online Wisdom Library curates the essential teachings of the living Himalayan Tradition. This offering is a unique counterpart to our in-person Mission Programs, empowering students by providing online learning resources to enrich their study and practice outside the classroom.

Our online Wisdom Library features multimedia blog content, livestreams, podcasts, yoga classes, meditation and relaxation practices, wellness content, and downloadable practice resources. These teachings capture our Mission Faculty's decades of study, practice, and teaching experience, featuring new content as well as the timeless teachings of Swami Rama and Pandit Rajmani Tigunait. We invite seekers and students of the Himalayan Tradition to become a Himalayan Institute Mission Member, which grants unlimited access to the Wisdom Library. Mission Membership supports the Institute's global humanitarian efforts, while helping you deepen your study and practice in the living Himalayan Tradition.

Spiritual Excursions

Since 1972, the Himalayan Institute has been organizing pilgrimages throughout India and Nepal. Our spiritual excursions follow the traditional pilgrimage routes where adepts of the Himalayas lived and practiced. For thousands of years, pilgrimage has been an essential part of yoga sadhana, offering spiritual seekers the opportunity to experience the transformative power of living shrines of the Himalayan Tradition. Join us on pilgrimage in the Himalayas, or for retreat offerings at the Himalayan Institute Khajuraho campus in central India.

Global Humanitarian Projects

The Himalayan Institute's humanitarian mission is yoga in action—offering spiritually grounded healing and transformation to the world. Our humanitarian projects serve rural communities in India and Cameroon through education and literacy initiatives, health services, and vocational training. By putting yoga philosophy into practice, our programs are empowering communities globally with the knowledge and tools needed for a lasting social transformation at the grassroots level.

Publications

The Himalayan Institute publishes over 60 titles on yoga, philosophy, spirituality, science, ayurveda, and holistic health. These include the best-selling books *Living with the Himalayan Masters* and *The Science of Breath* by Swami Rama; *Vishoka Meditation, Sri Sukta*, and two commentaries on the *Yoga Sutra: The Secret of the Yoga Sutra: Samadhi Pada* and *The Practice of the Yoga Sutra: Sadhana Pada* by Pandit Rajmani Tigunait, PhD; and the award-winning *Yoga: Mastering the Basics* by Sandra Anderson and Rolf Sovik, PsyD. These books are for everyone: the interested reader, the spiritual novice, and the experienced practitioner.

PureRejuv Wellness Center

For over 40 years, the PureRejuv Wellness Center has fulfilled part of the Institute's mission to promote healthy and sustainable lifestyles. PureRejuv combines Eastern philosophy and Western medicine in an integrated approach to holistic health—nurturing balance and healing at home and at work. We offer the opportunity to find healing and renewal through on-site and online wellness retreats and individual wellness services, including therapeutic massage and bodywork, yoga therapy, ayurveda, biofeedback, natural medicine, and one-on-one consultations with our integrative medical staff.

Total Health Products

The Himalayan Institute, the developer of the original Neti Pot, manufactures a health line specializing in traditional and modern ayurvedic supplements and body care. We are dedicated to a holistic and sustainable lifestyle by providing products that use natural, non-GMO ingredients and eco-friendly packaging. Part of every purchase supports our global humanitarian projects, further developing and reinforcing our core mission of spirituality in action.

Residential Service Programs

Karma yoga (selfless service) is at the heart of the Institute's mission, and is embodied by the Himalayan Institute Residential Program and the SEVA Work-Study Program offered at our Honesdale campus. Learn more about residential service opportunities on our website, and join a vibrant community of practitioners dedicated to service.

For further information about our programs, humanitarian projects, and products:

call:	800-822-4547
email:	info@HimalayanInstitute.org
write:	Himalayan Institute 952 Bethany Turnpike Honesdale, PA 18431
or visit:	HimalayanInstitute.org

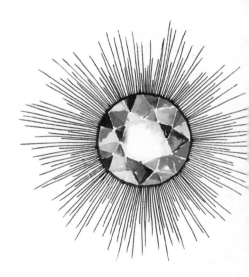

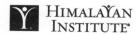

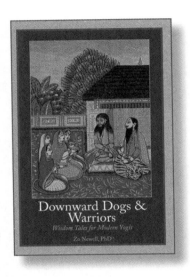

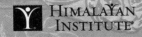